Methods in Molecular Biology

For further volumes:
http://www.springer.com/series/7651

Streptococcus pneumoniae

Methods and Protocols

Edited by

Federico Iovino

Department of Microbiology, Tumor and Cell Biology Karolinska Institutet, Bioclinicum, Stockholm, Sweden

Department of Clinical Microbiology, Karolinska University Hospital, Stockholm, Sweden

Humana Press

Editor
Federico Iovino
Department of Microbiology, Tumor and Cell Biology
Karolinska Institutet, Bioclinicum
Stockholm, Sweden

Department of Clinical Microbiology
Karolinska University Hospital
Stockholm, Sweden

ISSN 1064-3745 ISSN 1940-6029 (electronic)
Methods in Molecular Biology
ISBN 978-1-4939-9198-3 ISBN 978-1-4939-9199-0 (eBook)
https://doi.org/10.1007/978-1-4939-9199-0

Library of Congress Control Number: 2019934805

This Humana Press imprint is published by the registered company Springer Science+Business Media, LLC part of Springer Nature.
The registered company address is: 233 Spring Street, New York, NY 10013, U.S.A.

Aim of the Book

Abstract

The Gram-positive bacterium *Streptococcus pneumoniae*, the pneumococcus, is a leading cause of mortality and morbidity worldwide and considered a serious threat in today's public health. It is a major contributor of severe diseases such as pneumonia and bacteremia and the main etiological cause of bacterial meningitis. All these diseases are defined as invasive pneumococcal disease (IPD). Even though pneumococci can cause invasive diseases, *S. pneumoniae* is a commensal, and in fact, it normally colonizes the nasopharyngeal epithelium asymptomatically. In the last decade, there have been important advances in the development of new methodologies to study the cell biology of the pneumococcus and how *S. pneumoniae* interacts with the human host. The aim of this book is to shed light into the materials and methods used to study pneumococci and IPD.

Key words: *Streptococcus pneumoniae* • Pneumococcus • Host • Molecular biology • Methods

Federico Iovino

Preface

The Gram-positive bacterium *Streptococcus pneumoniae*, the pneumococcus, is considered a serious threat in today's public health, not only because it is a major cause of serious diseases like pneumonia, bacteremia, and meningitis but also because of the overuse and misuse of antibiotics; the cases of antibiotic resistance have increased dramatically [1–4]. In addition, introduction of the pneumococcal conjugate vaccines (PCVs) has decreased the incidence of pneumococcal meningitis caused by the 7 (PCV7) or 13 (PCV13) serotypes included in the vaccine, but the incidence of invasive pneumococcal disease caused by non-vaccine types has increased [5, 6].

Nowadays, there have been important advances in many techniques used to study the molecular biology of the pneumococcus, from the methodologies to study protein and gene expression to novel experimental setups to study invasive pneumococcal disease in vivo. Importantly, in the recent years, new discoveries, like the CRISPR/Cas9 system, have had a tremendous impact in biomedical research. Imaging techniques have grown tremendously in the recent years; today, the molecular mechanisms regulating the cell biology of the pneumococcus and bacterial interaction with the human host can be investigated with high-, through live-cell imaging, and super-resolution microscopy. Last but not least, epidemiological studies have become more and more comprehensive and accurate, thanks to the extensive use of whole-genome sequencing and the availability of collections from many countries and international research consortia of bacterial clinical isolates.

Materials and methods are the bridge that consent scientists to verify hypotheses, collect results, and create knowledge. The aim of this book is to shed light into all the methods, materials, equipment, and new technologies developed and used nowadays to study the cell biology of the pneumococcus, at a protein and gene level, the pneumococcal interaction with the human host, both in vitro and in vivo, and the epidemiology of IPD. Essentially, each chapter aims to describe a specific technique or application in an easy-to-follow step-by-step format for the scientific community.

Karolinska Institutet
Stockholm, Sweden

Federico Iovino

References

1. Laxminarayan R, Duse A, Wattal C (2013) Antibiotic resistance-the need for global solutions. Lancet Infect Dis 13:1057–98
2. Dockrell DH, Whyte MKB, Mitchell TJ (2012) Pneumococcal pneumonia: mechanisms of infection and resolution. Chest 142:482–491

3. O'Brien KL, Wolfson LJ, Watt JP (2009) Hib and pneumococcal global burden of disease study team, burden of disease caused by streptococcus pneumoniae in children younger than 5 years: global estimates. Lancet 374:893–902
4. van de Beek, D, de Gans J, Tunkel AR (2006) Community-acquired bacterial meningitis in adults. N Engl J Med 354:44–53
5. Browall S, Backhaus E, Naucler P (2014) Clinical manifestations of invasive pneumococcal disease by vaccine and non-vaccine types. Eur Respir J 44:1646–57
6. Galanis I, Lindstrand A, Darenberg J (2016) Effects of PCV7 and PCV13 on invasive pneumococcal disease and carriage in Stockholm, Sweden. Eur Respir J 47:1208–1218

Contents

Part IV The Proteome and Proteomics of *Streptococcus pneumoniae*

Part V *Streptococcus pneumoniae*-Host Interactions: In Vitro and In Vivo Models

Part VI Public Health, Epidemiology, and Biostatistics

Contributors

SURYA D. AGGARWAL • *Department of Biological Sciences, Carnegie Mellon University, Pittsburgh, PA, USA*
MATHIEU A. BERGÉ • *Laboratoire de Microbiologie et Génétique Moléculaires (LMGM), Centre de Biologie Intégrative (CBI), Toulouse, France; Centre National de la Recherche Scientifique (CNRS), Université de Toulouse, Université Paul Sabatier (UPS), Toulouse, France*
CAROLINE BERGENFELZ • *Wallenberg Laboratory, Division of Experimental Infection Medicine, Department of Translational Medicine, Lund University, Malmö, Sweden*
TERRY BRISSAC • *Department of Microbiology, School of Medicine, The University of Alabama at Birmingham, Birmingham, AL, USA*
NATHALIE CAMPO • *Laboratoire de Microbiologie et Génétique Moléculaires (LMGM), Centre de Biologie Intégrative (CBI), Toulouse, France; Centre National de la Recherche Scientifique (CNRS), Université de Toulouse, Université Paul Sabatier (UPS), Toulouse, France*
YASHUAN CHAO • *Wallenberg Laboratory, Division of Experimental Infection Medicine, Department of Translational Medicine, Lund University, Malmö, Sweden*
KEDING CHENG • *National Microbiology Laboratory, Public Health Agency of Canada, Winnipeg, MB, Canada; Department of Human Anatomy and Cell Sciences, College of Medicine, University of Manitoba, Winnipeg, MB, Canada*
HUIXIA CHUAN • *Henan Center for Disease Control and Prevention, Zhengzhou, Henan, People's Republic of China*
MARÍA DOLORES CIMA-CABAL • *Escuela Superior de Ingeniería y Tecnología (ESIT), Universidad Internacional de La Rioja (UNIR), Logroño, Spain*
ROLANDO A. CUEVAS • *Department of Biological Sciences, Carnegie Mellon University, Pittsburgh, PA, USA*
JUAN R. DE LOS TOYOS • *Área de Inmunología, Facultad de Medicina y Ciencias de la Salud, Universidad de Oviedo, Oviedo, Spain*
MARÍA DEL MAR GARCÍA-SUÁREZ • *Escuela Superior de Ingeniería y Tecnología (ESIT), Universidad Internacional de La Rioja (UNIR), Logroño, Spain*
RORY A. EUTSEY • *Department of Biological Sciences, Carnegie Mellon University, Pittsburgh, PA, USA*
NORMAN K. FRY • *Immunisation and Countermeasures Division, National Infection Service, Public Health England, London, UK; Respiratory and Vaccine Preventable Bacterial Reference Unit (RVPBRU), National Infection Service Laboratories, Public Health England, London, UK*
SANTIAGO F. GONZALEZ • *Institute for Research in Biomedicine, Università della Svizzera italiana, Bellinzona, Switzerland*
ANDERS P. HAKANSSON • *Wallenberg Laboratory, Division of Experimental Infection Medicine, Department of Translational Medicine, Lund University, Malmö, Sweden*
SVEN HAMMERSCHMIDT • *Department of Molecular Genetics and Infection Biology, Interfaculty Institute for Genetics and Functional Genomics, University of Greifswald, Greifswald, Germany*

Birgitta Henriques-Normark • *Department of Microbiology, Tumor and Cell Biology, Karolinska Institutet, Bioclinicum, Stockholm, Sweden; Department of Clinical Microbiology, Karolinska University Hospital, Stockholm, Sweden; Singapore Centre on Environmental Life Sciences Engineering (SCELSE), Lee Kong Chian School of Medicine (LKC), Nanyang Technological University (NTU), Singapore, Singapore*

N. Luisa Hiller • *Department of Biological Sciences, Carnegie Mellon University, Pittsburgh, PA, USA*

Federico Iovino • *Department of Microbiology, Tumor and Cell Biology, Karolinska Institutet, Bioclinicum, Stockholm, Sweden; Department of Clinical Microbiology, Karolinska University Hospital, Stockholm, Sweden*

Morten Kjos • *Faculty of Chemistry, Biotechnology and Food Science, Norwegian University of Life Sciences, Ås, Norway*

Shamez N. Ladhani • *Paediatric Infectious Diseases Research Group, Institute for Infection and Immunity, St. George's, University of London, London, UK; Immunisation and Countermeasures Division, National Infection Service, Public Health England, London, UK*

Cushla McGoverin • *Department of Physics, The University of Auckland, Auckland, New Zealand; The Dodd-Walls Centre for Photonic and Quantum Technologies, Auckland, New Zealand*

Isabelle Mortier-Barrière • *Laboratoire de Microbiologie et Génétique Moléculaires (LMGM), Centre de Biologie Intégrative (CBI), Toulouse, France; Centre National de la Recherche Scientifique (CNRS), Université de Toulouse, Université Paul Sabatier (UPS), Toulouse, France*

Godwin Oligbu • *Paediatric Infectious Diseases Research Group, Institute for Infection and Immunity, St. George's, University of London, London, UK; Immunisation and Countermeasures Division, National Infection Service, Public Health England, London, UK*

Carlos J. Orihuela • *Department of Microbiology, School of Medicine, The University of Alabama at Birmingham, Birmingham, AL, USA*

Fang Ou • *Department of Physics, The University of Auckland, Auckland, New Zealand; The Dodd-Walls Centre for Photonic and Quantum Technologies, Auckland, New Zealand*

Miguel Palomino-Segura • *Institute for Research in Biomedicine, Università della Svizzera italiana, Bellinzona, Switzerland; Graduate School of Cellular and Molecular Sciences, Faculty of Medicine, University of Bern, Bern, Switzerland*

Patrice Polard • *Laboratoire de Microbiologie et Génétique Moléculaires (LMGM), Centre de Biologie Intégrative (CBI), Toulouse, France; Centre National de la Recherche Scientifique (CNRS), Université de Toulouse, Université Paul Sabatier (UPS), Toulouse, France*

Marc Prudhomme • *Laboratoire de Microbiologie et Génétique Moléculaires (LMGM), Centre de Biologie Intégrative (CBI), Toulouse, France; Centre National de la Recherche Scientifique (CNRS), Université de Toulouse, Université Paul Sabatier (UPS), Toulouse, France*

Manfred Rohde • *Central Facility for Microscopy, HZI—Helmholtz Centre for Infection Research, Braunschweig, Germany*

Vicky Sender • *Department of Microbiology, Tumor and Cell Biology, Karolinska Institutet, Bioclinicum, Stockholm, Sweden*

Adam Sierakowiak • *Department of Oncology-Pathology, Karolinska Institutet, Stockholm, Sweden*

ANGELA SLOAN • *National Microbiology Laboratory, Public Health Agency of Canada, Winnipeg, MB, Canada*
NORMA SUÁREZ • *Department of Biotechnology, Faculty of Medicine, Institute of Hygiene, University of the Republic, Montevideo, Uruguay*
SIMON SWIFT • *School of Medical Sciences, The University of Auckland, Auckland, New Zealand*
ESTHER TEXEIRA • *Department of Biotechnology, Faculty of Medicine, Institute of Hygiene, University of the Republic, Montevideo, Uruguay*
RAYMOND TSANG • *National Microbiology Laboratory, Public Health Agency of Canada, Winnipeg, MB, Canada*
FRÉDÉRIQUE VANHOLSBEECK • *Department of Physics, The University of Auckland, Auckland, New Zealand; The Dodd-Walls Centre for Photonic and Quantum Technologies, Auckland, New Zealand*
FERNANDO VAZQUEZ • *Departamento de Microbiología, Hospital Universitario Central de Asturias & Fundación para la Investigación y la Innovación Biosanitaria del Principado de Asturias (FINBA), Oviedo, Spain; Departamento de Biología Funcional & Ophthalmology, Vision Sciences and Advanced Therapies Research Group, Instituto Universitario Fernández-Vega, Universidad de Oviedo, Oviedo, Spain*
JONI WHITE • *The Dodd-Walls Centre for Photonic and Quantum Technologies, Auckland, New Zealand; School of Medical Sciences, The University of Auckland, Auckland, New Zealand*
CAROL A. WOOLFORD • *Department of Biological Sciences, Carnegie Mellon University, Pittsburgh, PA, USA*
LU ZHANG • *Henan Center for Disease Control and Prevention, Zhengzhou, Henan, People's Republic of China*
JIANWEI ZHOU • *National Microbiology Laboratory, Public Health Agency of Canada, Winnipeg, MB, Canada*

About the Editor

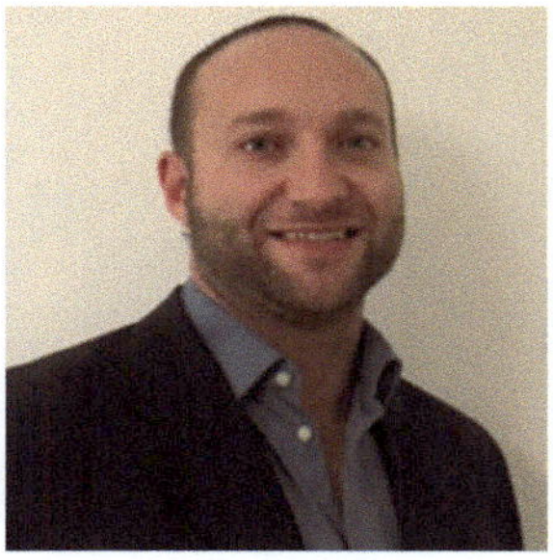

Federico Iovino has studied Biological Sciences, bachelor's and master's, at the University of Pavia in Italy. After his undergraduate studies, he moved to the University Medical Center of Groningen, the Netherlands, to perform his PhD in Medical Microbiology under the supervision of Prof. Jan Maarten van Dijl and Prof. Grietje Molema, studying how *Streptococcus pneumoniae* interacts with endothelial cells causing invasive pneumococcal disease, in particular meningitis. After his PhD graduation in November 2013, he immediately started his postdoc in December 2013 at the Karolinska Institutet in the laboratory of Prof. Birgitta Henriques-Normark where he continued his studies on pneumococcal meningitis. Federico's postdoc studies have been published in leading international journals like the *Journal of Clinical Investigation*, the *Journal of Experimental Medicine*, the *Journal of Infectious Diseases*, and *Trends in Microbiology.*

Federico Iovino is currently Assistant Professor at the Karolinska Institutet. His team conducts research focused on studying how bacterial pathogens after translocation across the blood-brain barrier interact with the different cell types of the brain (astrocytes, pericytes, neurons and microglia).

Part I

Cultivation of *Streptococcus pneumoniae* In Vitro

Chapter 1

Optimal Conditions for *Streptococcus pneumoniae* Culture: In Solid and Liquid Media

Norma Suárez and Esther Texeira

Abstract

Control of *Streptococcus pneumoniae* is mainly achieved by the use of existing vaccines. Capsular polysaccharides are the major antigenic component and are also the main virulence factor.

Capsular polysaccharides must fulfill requirements of purity, uniformity, and an accurate molecular weight to be used as vaccine antigens. Vaccine production largely relies on cultivation of the pathogen in appropriate conditions.

Here we describe widely used techniques to culture *S. pneumoniae* based on solid or complex liquid media, which are successfully applied in the diagnosis of the pathogen and in development and production of *S. pneumoniae* vaccines. Furthermore, we present a new chemically defined medium that can be used at lab scale.

Key words *S. pneumoniae*, Cultivation media, Chemically defined media (CDM)

1 Introduction

Laboratory diagnosis and treatment of invasive diseases caused by *S. pneumoniae* (e.g., otitis, pneumonia, and meningitis) rely on its recognition and identification. This initially begins with the cultivation of the microorganism in different culture media known worldwide [1–3]. Cultivation of the microorganism is also needed for the production of capsular polysaccharides, the main component of *S. pneumoniae* vaccines [4–7].

Several cultivation media are known for this organism. Solid and liquid agar (Luria Broth Agar) are the most common semisolid media for bacterial culture. (Agar is a hydrocolloid derived from red algae capable of remaining liquid until cooled to 40 degrees, the temperature at which it gels.) Agar is supplemented with defibrinated blood because of the bacteria's high metabolic requirement. Sheep, horse, and pig blood are used, as well as human blood-agar (HuBA) which is widely used in developing countries [8–12].

Federico Iovino (ed.), *Streptococcus pneumoniae: Methods and Protocols*, Methods in Molecular Biology, vol. 1968, https://doi.org/10.1007/978-1-4939-9199-0_1,

Tryptic soy broth or Todd Hewitt broth are among the best-known liquid media frequently recommended for the cultivation of fastidious organisms or to culture *S. pneumoniae* to obtain the serotype specific capsular polysaccharides used as antigens for vaccine production. They are supplemented with yeast extract, or other sources of carbon and nitrogen. These sources may be of vegetable origin and are widely used in vaccine production [2, 13, 14].

According to good manufacturing practices (GMP), the medium used to produce vaccine antigens must contain only essential components that allow maximum cell density and the reproducibility of the process. Chemically defined media are of value in studying the minimal nutritional requirements of microorganisms. Texeira and collaborators have recently proposed a new chemically defined medium for the cultivation of *S. pneumoniae* serotype 1 in order to achieve a high purity product, reduce the number of adverse reactions caused by complex media, and meet preestablished standards at all stages of the vaccine production process [11]. However, complex media are still the cultivation technique of choice for large-scale production because of the yield obtained and the lower production costs.

In this chapter we describe useful techniques for culturing *S. pneumoniae* both on solid and in liquid media.

2 Materials

Deionized water is preferred for preparing solutions. All the reagents may be stored at room temperature, except ovine blood, which should be stored at 4 °C for a period no longer than 10 days.

3 Methods

3.1 Culture of S. pneumoniae on Solid Medium

Medium preparation:

1. Dissolve 30 g of LBA powder in 1 l of deionized water (*see* **Note 1**).
2. Heat up to boiling point and separate the solution into 200 ml glass bottles.
3. Sterilize the bottles at 121 °C and store them at room temperature.

3.2 LBA–Blood Preparation

1. Take one of previously prepared LBA flasks and heat the solution until melting it (*see* **Note 2**).
2. Add 20 ml of sterile ovine blood, mix gently, and pour 20 ml into 10 petri dishes (*see* **Notes 3** and **4**).

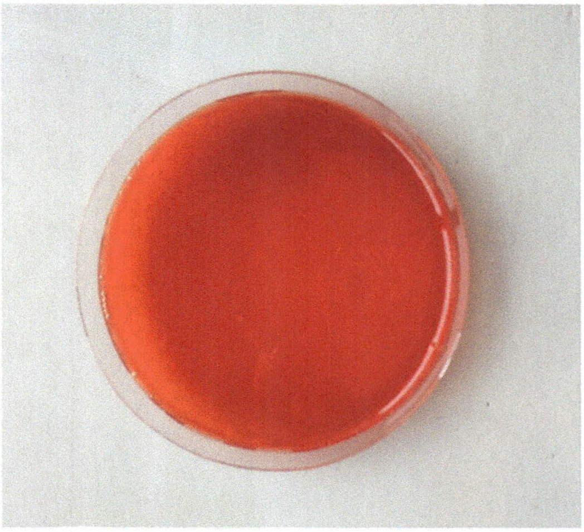

Fig. 1 Ovine blood agar plate. A sterile ovine blood agar plate after being at 37 °C overnight; no bacteria growth is observed

3. Cover the plates, let them cool, and place them at 37 °C overnight.
4. Take out the plates. If no growth is observed then the plates are ready to be used or stored at 2–8 °C until they are required Fig. 1.

3.3 Inoculation of Strain onto the LBA Plate

1. Take a cryotube with the selected strain of *S. pneumoniae* (*see* **Note 5**).
2. Defrost quickly under tap water.
3. Take a loop of the strain and seed it over the surface of the plate.
4. Refreeze the remaining content of the cryotube.
5. Incubate the inoculated plate at 37 °C in 5% CO_2 for 16–20 h.
6. At the end of the incubation time, the morphology and size of the colony are observed and Gram staining is done to observe the microscopic characteristics (Fig. 2) (*See* **Note 6**).

3.4 Preparation of TSB Vegetable Complex Media

Prepare 1 l of tryptic soy broth (TSB) medium by dissolving the quantity recommended by the manufacturers and then autoclaving for 15 min at 121 °C [15].

3.5 Preparation of Chemically Defined Media

The preparation of 1 l of defined media is a multistep procedure which includes the prior preparation of a number of solutions, such as basal medium solution, solutions of vitamins, salts, and growth factors, and a sodium bicarbonate/thioglycolic acid solution.

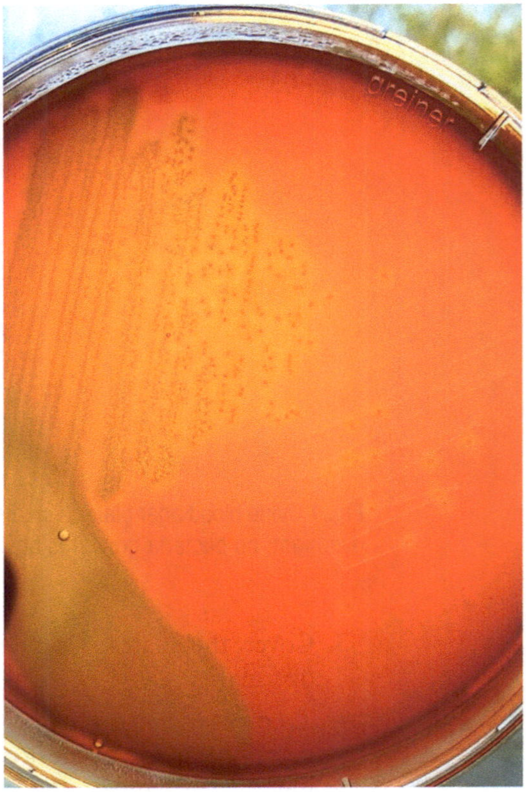

Fig. 2 *S. pneumoniae* colony morphology. *Streptococcus pneumoniae* colonies appearance after cultivation on *blood agar* in 5% CO_2, overnight. Colonies are surrounded by zones of alpha-hemolysis

1. Prepare 1 l of basal media by weighing out amino acids 35 mg/l L-tryptophan, 65 mg/l glycine, 166 mg/l L-cystine,; 144 mg/l L-tyrosine, 230 mg/l L-lysine, 173 mg/l L-valine, 230 mg/l L-leucine, 170 mg/l L-isoleucine, 120 mg/l L-threonine, 73 mg/l L-methionine, 184 mg/l L-aspartic acid, 43 m/l L-proline, 55 mg/l L-histidine hydrochloride, 125 mg/l L-arginine hydrochloride, 125 mg/l L-phenylalanine, 235 mg/l L-serine. Add to the solution monobasic potassium phosphate, monobasic sodium phosphate, and dibasic sodium phosphate (5.5, 3.2, and 7.3 g respectively).
2. Prepare vitamins solution dissolving the components in distilled water: 0.15 mg/ml biotin, 100 mg/ml nicotinic acid, 100 mg/ml pyridoxal, 500 mg/ml calcium pantothenate, 100 mg/ml thiamine, 100 mg/ml riboflavin, 1000 mg/ml adenine sulfate, 1000 mg/ml uracil. The solution must be aliquoted and maintained at −20 °C (*see* **Note 7**).
3. Prepare a salt solution dissolving the components (g/l) in distilled water: 250 g/l magnesium sulfate $7H_2O$, 2.5 g/l

ferrous sulfate $7H_2O$, 0.4 g/l zinc sulfate $7H_2O$, 0.2 g/l manganese sulfate. Add 10 ml 0.1 M chlorhydric acid.

4. Prepare a growth factors solution by adding to 200 ml of the vitamin solution (3), and 40 ml of the salt solution (4) the growth factors L-glutamine, asparagine, and choline chlorhydrate in the following amounts, 12.5 g, 2 g, and 0.2 g respectively.
5. Prepare a sodium bicarbonate ($NaHCO_3$) and thioglycolic acid solution as follows:
6. 1 g of $NaHCO_3$ and 1 ml of thioglycolic acid (80%) mixed in 25 ml of distilled water. This unstable mixture is prepared and immediately added to the medium prior to sterilization.
7. Prepare 1 l of defined medium as follows: 900 ml basal medium, 50 ml of vitamin, salt, and growth factor solution (5), 12.5 g of glucose, and 25 ml bicarbonate/thioglycolic acid solution and complete the volume with distilled water.
8. Adjust the pH to 7.2.
9. Filter the solution through Whatman filter paper No. 2 to remove large impurities and sterilize by filtration through a 0.22 μm-pore size membrane.
10. Place at 37 °C in 5% CO_2 atmosphere overnight (*see* **Note 8**).

3.6 Inoculum Preparation and Culture

1. Take aliquots of a frozen tube of the strain of *S. pneumoniae* to be cultured.
2. Seed 3– 5 tubes containing 10 ml each of TSB vegetable medium.
3. Culture at 37 °C with 5% CO_2 until a cell density of approximately 7×10^9 cells/ml is attained (based on McFarland's scale) (*see* **Note 9**).
4. Use the contents of one of those tubes as the inoculum to seed a 1 l flask.
5. Culture *S. pneumoniae* in a 5% CO_2 atmosphere for 16–24 h in the selected liquid medium (TSB or chemically defined medium) Fig. 3.
6. Check the purity of the culture by Gram stain and view the capsule of *S. pneumoniae* by a Quellung reaction at the microscope Fig. 4 [16].
7. Inactivate culture growth with 0.09% sodium azide.

4 Notes

1. Luria broth is a nutritionally rich medium recommended for the culture of various microorganisms. Follow the preparation procedures as directed by the manufacturer [9].

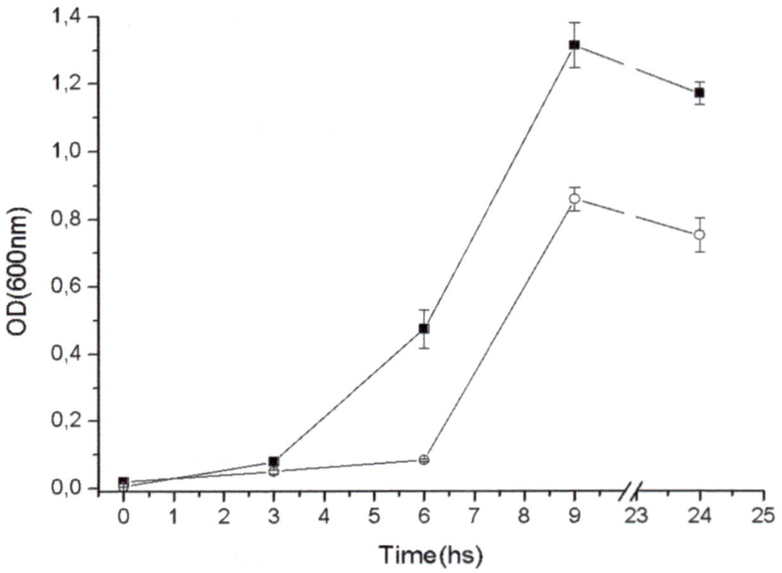

Fig. 3 Growth profile of *S. pneumoniae* in TSB (○) and in CDM (■). *S. pneumoniae* is capable of grow in either commercially available media (TSB) or chemically defined medium (CDM). The use of CDM medium is a change in usual cultivation techniques

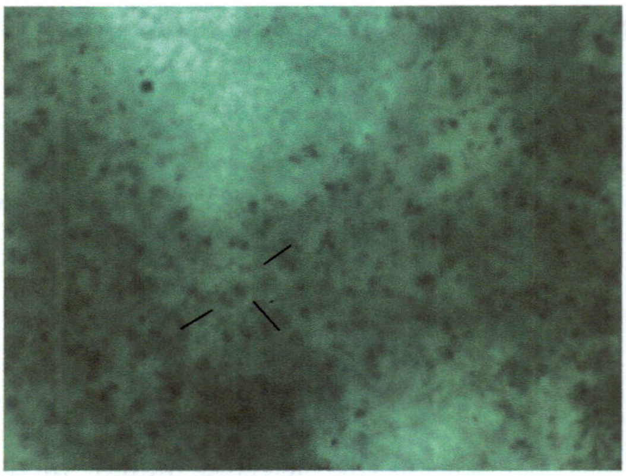

Fig. 4 Microscopic view of the capsule of *S. pneumoniae.* Capsule of *S. pneumoniae* were viewed at the microscope under 100× magnification in a Quellung reaction (black stripe)

2. Melt the LBA solution in a microwave oven at 40% potency for 5–8 min. Allow the medium to cool until it can be handled, that is, until you can keep your hand around the flask and it feels OK to touch it (approximately 45 °C).
3. Check the sterility of the blood to be used by cultivation for 24 h in thioglycolate and T-Broth for the differentiation of

anaerobic or aerobic contaminant microorganisms. At the end of this time no bacterial growth should be observed.

4. To avoid the formation of water drops over the surface of the medium, you must flame the loops gently with a Bunsen burner.
5. These procedures may be done in the laminar flow cabinet. Generally, most serotypes of *S. pneumoniae* are grown in commercially available media; the chemically defined medium has been tested in a considerable number of *S. pneumoniae* serotypes suggesting that almost all serotypes will grow without any problem in the chemically defined medium.
6. *S. pneumoniae* morphology presents a colony size of 1–2 mm diameter, white, with alfa hemolysis and central depression due to autolysis.
7. The vitamin solution can be prepared in smaller volumes and stored at a temperature of −20 °C for up to 2 months.
8. The medium solution must be transparent at the end of this time.
9. The comparison of the culture with the McFarland's scale must be done by eye.

References

1. InstitutMerieux. (1980) Procédé de purification de polyosides de *Streptococcus pneumoniae* et vaccin à base de polyosides ainsi purifiés Brevet Belge No. 8026320
2. Kim SN, Min KK, Choi HI, Kim SW, Pio SN, Rhee DK (1996) Optimization of culture conditions for production of pneumococcal capsular polysacharide type IV. Arch Pharm Res 19(3):173–177
3. Massaldi H, Besssio MI, Suarez N, Texeira E, Rossi S, Ferreira F (2010) Features of bacterial growth and polysaccharide production of *Streptococcus pneumoniae* serotype 14. Biotechnol Appl Biochem 55:37–43. https://doi.org/10.1042/BA20090218
4. Leal MM, Pereira DSG, Jessouroun E, Couto MAPG, Pereira N (2001) Investigation of cultivation conditions for capsular polysaccharide production by *Streptococcus pneumoniae* serotype 14. Electron J 14:1–7. https://doi.org/10.2225/vol14-issue5-fulltext-6
5. Tarahomjoo S, Jalali M (2015) Investigation of appropriate cultivation approach for capsular polysaccharide production by *Streptococcus pneumoniae* serotype 19 American journal of. Microbiol Res 3(6):197–200. https://doi.org/10.12691/ajmr-3-6-4.
6. Suárez N, Franco Fraguas L, Ferreira F, Massaldi M (2008) Improved conjugation and purification strategies for the preparation of protein polysaccharide conjugates. J Chromatogr A 1213:169–175. https://doi.org/10.1016/j.chroma.2008.10.030
7. Suárez N (2016) Optimal conditions for *Streptococcus pneumoniae* culture and for polysaccharide production for vaccines. Biol Med 8 (6). https://doi.org/10.4172/0974-8369.1000321
8. Hoeprich PO (1957) Evaluation of an improved chemically defined medium for the culture of *Diplococcus pneumoniae.* J Bacteriol 74:587–590
9. Luria SE, Burrous JW (1957) Hybridization between Escherichia Coli and Shigella. J Bacteriol 74:461–476
10. Russell FM, Biribo SSN, Selvaraj G, Oppedisano F, Warren S, Seduadua A, Mulholland EK, Carapetis JR (2006) As a bacterial culture medium, citrated sheep blood agar is a practical alternative to citrated human blood agar in Laboratories of Developing Countries. J Clin Microbiol 44(9):3346–3351. https://doi.org/10.1128/JCM.02631-05

11. Texeira E, Checa J, Rial A, Chabalgoity JA, Suárez N (2015) A new chemically defined medium for cultivation of *Streptococcus pneumoniae* serotype 1. J Biotech Res 6:54–62. ISSN: 1944-3285
12. Van De Rijn I, Kessler E (1980) Growth characteristics of group a streptococci in a new chemically defined medium. Infect Immun 27 (2):444–448
13. Hewitt LF, Todd EW (1932) A new culture medium for the production of antigenic streptococcal hæmolysin. J Pathol Bacteriol 35 (1):973–974
14. McCullough NB (1949) Laboratory tests in the diagnosis of brucellosis. Am J Public Health Nations Health 39:866–869
15. Murray PR, Baron EJ, Pfaller MA, Tenover FC, Yolken RH (1999) Manual of clinical microbiology, 7th edn. American Society for Microbiology, Washington, DC
16. Neufeld F (1902) Über die Agglutination der Pneumokokken und über die Theorien der Agglutination. Z Hyg Infekt 40:54–72

Part II

Microscopy Techniques to Study the Biology of *Streptococcus pneumoniae* and Pneumococcal Interactions with the Host

Chapter 2

Electron Microscopy to Study the Fine Structure of the Pneumococcal Cell

Sven Hammerschmidt and Manfred Rohde

Abstract

Electron microscopy allows for studying bacterial ultrastructure at high resolutions. Two types of electron microscopes are used for this purpose. The transmission electron microscope allows for access to inner bacterial ultrastructure when imaging ultrathin sections as well as cell wall-attached structures by negative staining, whereas scanning electron microscopy allows for the detection of structures on the bacterial cell surface alone or to study the interplay between pneumococci and their host cells. This chapter deals with recommendations for well-adapted methodologies to examine pneumococcal ultrastructure in detail. Especially, we focus on the preservation of the pneumococcal capsular polysaccharide, which represents an important virulence factor of pneumococci. Since capsules are highly hydrated structures, the introduction of a new fixation protocol involving lysine acetate, ruthenium red, and osmium (LRR fixation) results in a very well-preserved capsular structure in such a way that the amount of capsular material bound on the bacterial surface can be compared within different serotypes. In our method, capsular ultrastructure is preserved without the need for serotype-specific antibodies, which have been used in other studies to preserve the pneumococcal capsule. In addition, the new LRR fixation allows for studying the presence or absence of capsular material during adhesion and invasion of pneumococci on epithelial or endothelial host cells in cell culture experiments.

Key words Pneumococci, Pneumococcal capsule, Transmission electron microscopy, Field emission scanning electron microscopy, Cryo-FESEM, LRR embedding, LRWhite resin, Critical point drying, Infection

1 Introduction

For a long time, transmission electron microscopy (TEM) has been applied for studying the morphology and ultrastructure of gram-positive bacteria with a variety of different embedding protocols [1–7]. Nevertheless, even today we are waiting for an embedding protocol that allows for preserving intracellular ultrastructural details as well as extracellular attached structures like a capsular polysaccharide (CPS) of all the different gram-positive bacteria under close-to-nature conditions with electron microscopy. The modern newly developed technique of cryo electron tomography

Federico Iovino (ed.), *Streptococcus pneumoniae: Methods and Protocols*, Methods in Molecular Biology, vol. 1968, https://doi.org/10.1007/978-1-4939-9199-0_2,

(CET) might be the method of choice; but CET has also some drawbacks, and the technique is restricted by the size of the bacteria. This is especially the case when bacteria which have a width of more than 0.3 μm have to be imaged [8].

The embedding protocols usually aim to preserve ultrastructural details, eliminate water in the samples, and introduce heavy metals for contrast in TEM studies [4]. Therefore, embedding procedures include chemical fixation with aldehydes, introduction of heavy metals, dehydration with acetone/ethanol, and embedding in suitable resins. All these preparations steps are a prerequisite to cope with the environmental conditions in an electron microscope, especially with high vacuum and bombardment with high-energy electrons for imaging. Thus, it is obvious that these harsh treatments of the samples might not result in a proper preservation of the native ultrastructure of bacteria, in particular for those delicate structures like a bacterial glycocalyx. Nevertheless, by the introduction of special compounds it was possible to reveal overwhelming information about gram-positive bacterial ultrastructure. Especially the preservation of bacterial surface attached components like the bacterial capsule remains a major problem, because the preservation of these highly hydrated structures is a great challenge for electron microscopists [9].

The capsular polysaccharide of pneumococci surrounds this human pathobiont and is recognized as the sine qua non of virulence [10]. The variation of the CPS is high, and, to date, over 98 serotypes have been identified differing in their chemical composition of the CPS [10, 11]. Serotype-specific antibodies are used to distinguish serologically pneumococcal serotypes. The CPS is present in most strains and serotypes covalently attached to the peptidoglycan of pneumococci, and it is assumed that the LCP (LysR–Cps2A–Psr) protein family is involved in the attachment of these anionic polymers to the peptidoglycan [12]. The CPS is important to escape phagocytosis, undergoes phase variation, and masks other virulence factors such as adhesins [13, 14]. The biosynthesis of the CPS occurs via the synthase-dependent or the Wzy-dependent mechanism [10]. Analysis of the genomes indicated that Wzy-dependent serotypes share a conserved locus structure located on the chromosome between the genes *dexB* and *aliA*. Each CPS locus starts with conserved genes *cpsA* to *cpsD* followed by serotype-specific genes [10].

The pneumococcal capsular polysaccharides consist of acidic components like glucuronic acid, *N*-acetylmannosaminuronic acid, *N*-acetylgalactosamine, phosphate groups, ribitol, or arabinitol, which can be often found as high molecular weight polymers. These saccharides often have *O*-acetyl, phosphoglycerol, and pyruvyl acetal substitutions located at various sites and hence, all these compounds have in common that they are negatively charged and highly hydrated. Successful preservation of such a highly hydrated glycocalyx cannot be achieved with conventional embedding methods including glutaraldehyde fixation, osmification, and dehydration with acetone and embedding in an epoxy or acrylate resins. Reasons for these observations are manifold like inadequate stabilization of the highly substituted and variable polysaccharide moieties and alteration of delicate ultrastructural features during aldehyde fixation. Furthermore, highly hydrated and fibrous anionic arrays of polymers are condensed, collapsed or distorted during dehydration, embedding, and polymerization, or these polymers are totally or partially lost depending on the embedding protocols. To overcome the drawbacks of classical fixation procedures protocols have been developed, which include binding of serotype-specific antibodies to the corresponding capsule for stabilization of the capsular ultrastructure. Nevertheless, visualization and illustration of the pneumococcal capsular without addition of antibodies remains a challenge. For adequate stabilization and addition of contrast one requires reagents, which react properly with the highly polymerized, substituted, and anionic charged polysaccharides and other negatively charged moieties in the capsule. On an ultrastructural level, ruthenium red has been the reagent of choice for visualization of anionic polysaccharides on the surface of animal cells, because it binds strongly to negatively charged components [13, 15–19].

Hence, existing embedding procedures including the binding of ruthenium-red to negatively charged moieties were modified and adjusted to preserve pneumococcal capsular polysaccharides of different serotypes [15, 16]. The embedding schedule was customized in a way that it enabled to compare CPS thicknesses during the infection process of eukaryotic cells in a cell culture assay and in in vivo experiments. In addition, the modified method was also adjusted for FESEM studies [13]. During the development of a modified protocol it became obvious that incubation with ruthenium red alone does not preserve the ultrastructure very well. The introduction of lysine salts, especially lysine acetate, as a CPS stabilizing agent, was successful. The precipitation of bound ruthenium red with osmium gave sufficient contrast of the stabilized capsule in ultrathin sections [13]. In FESEM studies the presence and absence of capsular material on the surface of pneumococci could be demonstrated during the invasion process. In sum, a very well-preserved pneumococcal capsule was achieved with the lysine–ruthenium red–osmium (LRR) method [13]. In addition, the LRR method was also shown to preserve the capsular structures of different serotypes of other gram-positive bacteria like *Streptococcus pyogenes* and *Streptococcus suis*.

2 Materials

Prepare all solutions with distillated water and analytical grade commercially available reagents. For osmium tetroxide and uranyl acetate, follow strictly the existing safety regulations.

2.1 Dissolving of Osmium

1. Purchase osmium tetroxide in a glass ampule.
2. Heat the glass ampule with warm water until the osmium tetroxide crystals melt and form a single liquid droplet.
3. Bring the ampule back to room temperature.
4. Wrap the glass ampule tightly in aluminum foil, smash the ampule, unwrap, and collect the single osmium tetroxide crystal in a fume hood.
5. Place the crystal in distilled water or the adequate buffer for dissolving to the desired concentration. Stock solution 5% aqueous osmium tetroxide, store in an airtight brown bottle.

2.2 Dissolving Uranyl Acetate

1. Add 0.4 g uranyl acetate to 10 mL of distilled water (*see* **Note 1**)
2. Stir at room temperature until uranyl acetate is dissolved.
3. Take the supernatant and fill into 1.5 or 2.0 mL safe lock tubes and store in the dark or fill into brown glass bottles
4. Before usage, centrifuge for 2 min at 15,700 × *g*.

2.3 Preparation of 25% Aqueous Formaldehyde

1. Add 25 g of paraformaldehyde powder in a beaker (*see* **Note 2**).
2. Add 85 mL distilled water.
3. Heat until approximately 60 °C with stirring.
4. Add dropwise 10 M sodium hydroxide solution until all paraformaldehyde powder is dissolved.
5. Fill with distilled water to 100 mL.
6. Let the solution cool down to room temperature and leave it for 2 days at room temperature.
7. Filter the solution through a filter paper.
8. Leave the filtered solution at room temperature.
9. Before usage of the formaldehyde solution centrifuge for 2 min at 15,700 × *g*.
10. Take the supernatant for preparing the fixation solution.

2.4 Dissolving of Ruthenium Red

1. Prepare a stock solution of 0.15% ruthenium red in 0.2 M cacodylate buffer; this solution is double concentrated (*see* **Note 3**).
2. Cacodylate buffer consists of 0.1 M cacodylate, 0.09 M sucrose, 0.01 M $MgCl_2$, 0.01 M $CaCl_2$, pH 6.9 as end concentration.

3. With stirring dissolve ruthenium red at room temperature, normally a light precipitate of nondissolvable ruthenium red will remain.
4. Take the supernatant for preparing the fixation solutions.

2.5 LRWhite Resin

1. The acrylic resin LRWhite resin has been developed by the London Resin Company, Reading, England (*see* **Note 4**).
2. The resin can be purchased through any EM supplier.
3. Purchase the hard grade formula of the resin.
4. Add the accelerator only in the last step of infiltration.

3 Methods

3.1 Negative Staining

Negative staining is a rapid, easy-to-perform, and very reliable and reproducible method for analyzing bacteria, phages, or enzyme molecules in TEM studies. The method takes advantage of the deposition of heavy metal atoms like uranyl on the air-dried sample. Since the contrast in TEM images is based on scattering of electrons the resulting TEM image represents a projection of the entire sample, which consists of a translucent part and a grey to dark part in the images due to the scattered electrons on the heavy metal atoms [20, 21].

3.1.1 Preparation of Carbon Film on Mica

1. Cut out a piece of mica with 3 × 3 cm with a scissor.
2. With the aid of a scalpel or a razor blade cleave the mica peace in the middle to gain a clean and even surface.
3. Place the mica with the newly cut side facing up in a petri dish and fix with tape and place in the carbon evaporation apparatus.
4. For obtaining uniform thin carbon films use carbon strings.
5. Carbon strings are evaporated by the carbon coater unit by passing an electric current through the double carbon strings.
6. The applied procedure and settings are based on the available carbon coater apparatus in the laboratory.
7. Carbon-coated mica is stored in a petri dish and sealed with Parafilm™ to avoid humidification.

3.1.2 Negative Staining with Carbon Film

A metal grid is giving support for the carbon film and the specimen. The grid consists of an electron opaque component, the bars, and an electron translucent part, the open area. The number of grid bars and percentage of open area is varying depending of the grid types used; usually, 100–400 mesh (lines/inch) grids are used. Most EM grids are made of copper because they are the cheapest. In addition, the copper mesh also conducts heat away from the support film and helps to prevent specimen movement due to thermal expansion [22].

1. Centrifuge the 4% aqueous uranyl acetate solution for 2 min at 15,700 × *g* (*see* **Note 1**).
2. Pipet 30–40 μL droplets of the sample, washing solution (TE buffer (10 mM TRIS, 2 mM EDTA, pH 6.9) and distilled water) and 4% uranyl acetate on a clean piece of Parafilm™.
3. Take care that a pronounced convex meniscus is always visible.
4. Cut out a square of 2 mm × 2 mm from the carbon-coated mica and hold the piece with sharp, pointed forceps at one end of the piece of mica.
5. Introduce the carbon-coated piece of mica at a 45° slowly into the sample solution. The carbon film will float off the mica and particles will start to adsorb to the carbon film. Part of the carbon film still has contact with the mica and is held in place by the forceps.
6. The floating time (approximately 15–45 s) of the carbon film on the sample solution depends on the number of particles in the solution.
7. Remove the piece of mica slowly from the sample solution, the carbon film will fall back into its original position.
8. Remove excess sample solution by blotting on filter paper, but do not blot totally dry.
9. Using the same procedure as described above transfer the carbon film onto TE-buffer and distilled water; always remove excess fluid by blotting on filter paper.
10. Completely float the carbon film onto the staining solution by moving the piece of mica under the surface of the staining solution drop; open the forceps and the piece of mica will fall to the bottom of the droplet.
11. Pick up the carbon film with the adsorbed specimen using a suitable 100% acetone cleaned mesh copper grid (A 300 square mesh grid is recommended).
12. Slightly press on the grid with the forceps to get better contact of the carbon film to the grid.
13. Pick up the grid perpendicular from the staining solution drop, turn it around and blot the staining solution from the grid with filter paper.
14. For this purpose put the filter paper at the edge of the grid and let the solution creep up the filter paper until it does not flow anymore. Then remove the filter paper immediately. Take care that the grid is not blotted totally dry. A shiny liquid layer of the staining solution should be visible under a light source.

15. Using this procedure one usually gets a gradient of shallow stain and deeper stain on the carbon film.
16. Air-dry the grid with the attached carbon film with the help of a warm light globe by placing the grid under the globe at a distance of 1–2 cm for 10–15 s.
17. Examine by TEM.

3.2 Binding of Cationic Gold-Nanoparticles on Pneumococcal Capsular Polysaccharides

Since pneumococcal CPS exhibits a strong negatively charged surface the binding of positively charged compounds results in a better stabilization of the CPS structure. Gold-nanoparticles coated with lysine (cationic gold-nanoparticles, cat-gold) are positively charged; therefore, cat-gold binds via electrostatic interactions like van der Waals forces to pneumococcal capsules (Fig. 1).

1. Centrifuge in the medium used for growing pneumococci to achieve a fluffy pellet.
2. Resuspend the pellet in cacodylate/HEPES buffer with pH 3.0 for 10 min (*see* **Note 3**).
3. Centrifuge to achieve a fluffy pellet.
4. Resuspend pellet in cacodylate/HEPES buffer with pH 3.0.
5. Add 10 nm or 15 nm cat-gold to the solution until the solution shows a slight pink color; this step guarantees that excess cat-gold is in the solution to cover all exposed negatively charged sites.
6. Incubate for 15 min and centrifuge.
7. Resuspend in cacodylate/HEPES buffer, pH 7.0.
8. Add formaldehyde to an end concentration of 1% and leave on ice for 30 min (*see* **Note 2**).
9. Wash with cacodylate/HEPES buffer.
10. Perform negative staining with the cat-gold stained samples.
11. Be aware that due to the pH shift in the protocol a certain percentage of pneumococci will be destroyed.

3.3 Lysine–Ruthenium Red–Osmium (LRR) Embedding Procedure

The LRR embedding protocol is based on three different fixation/washing procedures in which the first fixation step is the most crucial. Importantly, the first fixation step should not be longer than 20 min for preservation of the pneumococcal capsule, at least in our hands (Figs. 2 and 3).

1. Centrifuge the 0.15% ruthenium red cacodylate solution for 2 min at 15,700 × *g*.
2. Centrifuge the bacteria in the medium. Take care to use the lowest possible *g*-value to achieve a fluffy bacterial pellet.

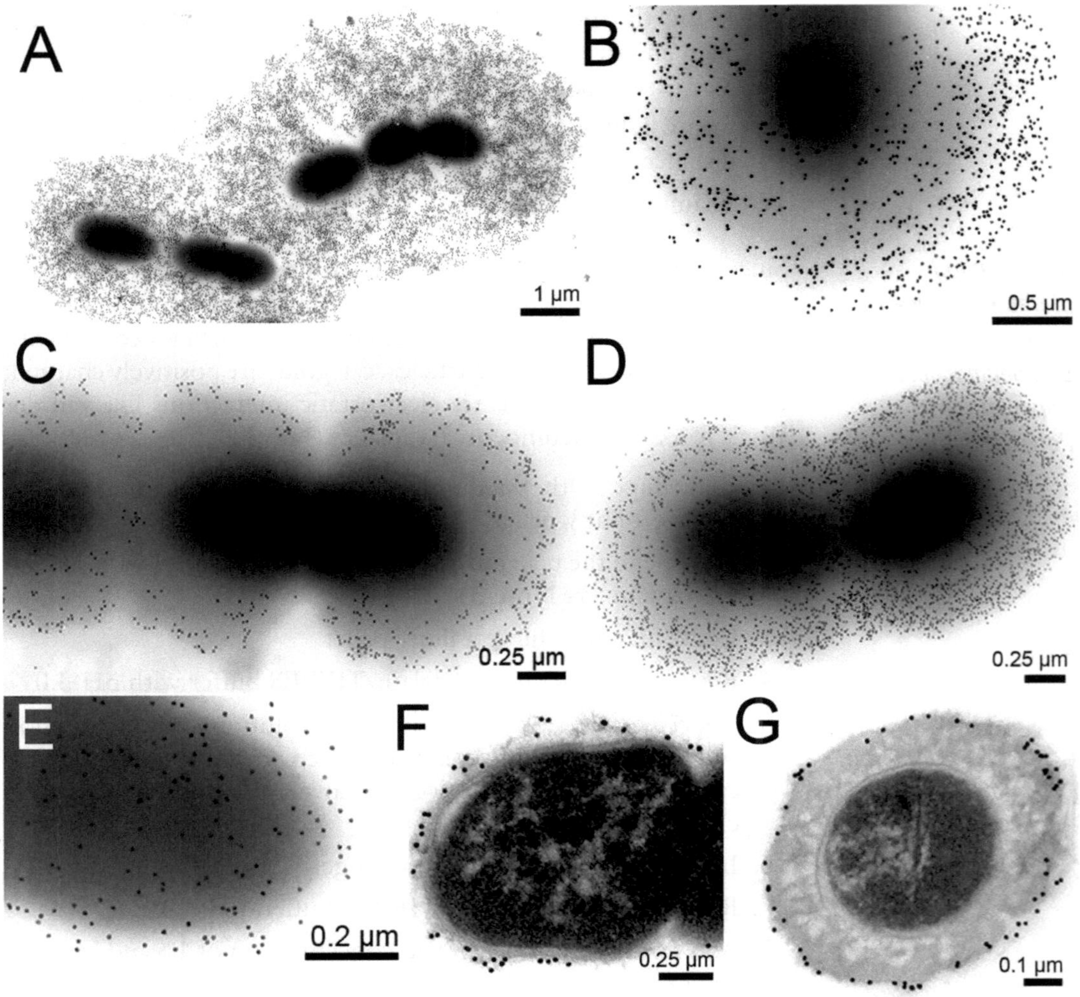

Fig. 1 Visualization of pneumococcal CPS applying cationic gold-nanoparticles. (**A**–**D**) Fixation of pneumococci in growth medium, pH shift to 3.0 with PBS followed by incubation with 1:75 diluted stock solution of 15 nm cationic gold-nanoparticles (**A**, **B**, **D**) or 1:200 diluted cationic gold-nanoparticles (**C**). (**E**) Fixation with glutaraldehyde destroys the capsular structure and cationic gold-nanoparticles bind only to the bacterial surface. (**A**–**E**) Negative staining with 0.5% uranyl acetate. (**F**) and (**G**) Ultrathin sections of glutardialdehyde- (**F**) and formaldehyde-fixed (**G**) pneumococci, after glutaraldehyde fixation capsular structures are lost, whereas in the formaldehyde-fixed sample, bound gold-nanoparticles at the edge of the capsule are detectable

3. Prepare fixation solution 1 per 1 mL volume: 0.5 mL of the 0.15% ruthenium red solution, 80 µL of the 25% formaldehyde solution, 100 µL of the 25% glutaraldehyde solution, 0.0155 g of lysine acetate; fill with distilled water to 1 mL.

   Very important: add the lysine acetate only immediately before usage of fixation solution 1 to the fixation solution.

4. Resuspend the fluffy bacteria pellet in fixation solution 1.

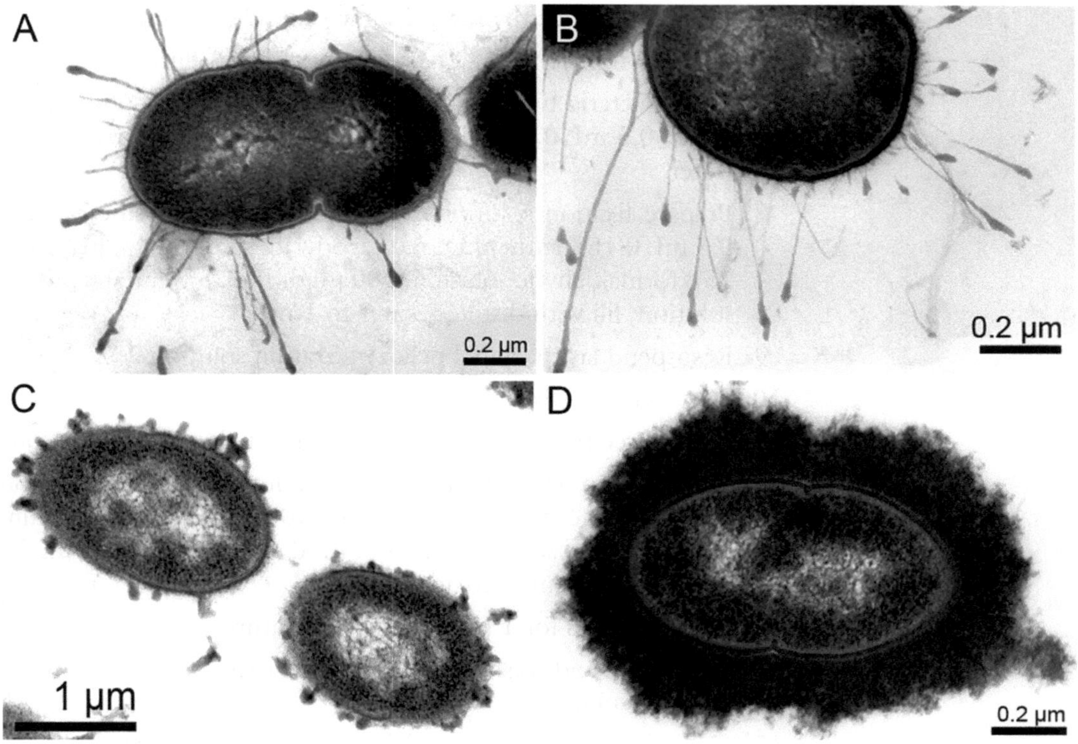

Fig. 2 Preservation of the pneumococcal capsule by lysine–ruthenium red–osmium fixation (LRR) and embedding in LRWhite resin. (**A**) and (**B**) Ultrathin sections of LRWhite embedded pneumococci demonstrate the loss of capsule after formaldehyde (**A**) and glutaraldehyde (**B**) fixation and embedding without stabilization of the capsule after acetone dehydration. (**C**) Incubation with ruthenium red prior to embedding keeps some capsular structures, dark material, on the pneumococcal surface. (**D**) Fixation following the LRR protocol shows full preservation of the pneumococcal capsule

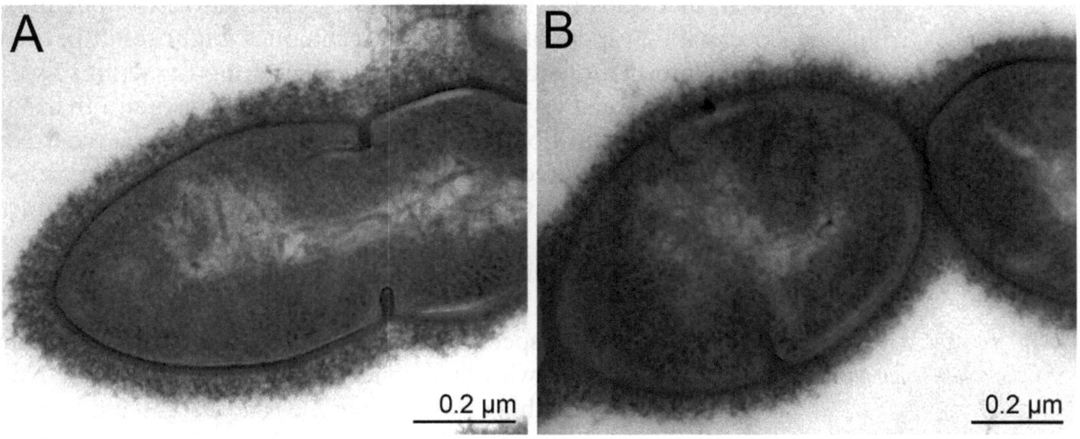

Fig. 3 Validation of the LRR fixation for preserving capsular ultrastructure in other streptococci (i.e., *Streptococcus suis*). (**A** and **B**) Two different clinical isolates of *S. suis* were fixed according to the LRR fixation protocol and embedded in LRWhite resin. Note the different sizes of the attached capsules of the two strains

5. Immediately put the sample on ice and fix for 20 min.
6. After 20 min centrifuge bacteria to achieve a fluffy pellet.
7. Wash bacteria twice with the following washing solution per 1 mL: 0.5 mL 0.15% ruthenium red solution, 0.5 mL distilled water,
8. Prepare fixation solution 2 per 1 mL without lysine acetate: 0.5 mL 0.15% ruthenium red cacodylate solution, 80 μL of the 25% formaldehyde solution, 100 μL of the 25% glutaraldehyde solution; fill with distilled water to 1 mL.
9. Resuspend last bacterial pellet in fixation solution 2.
10. Leave samples for 2 h on ice in fixation solution 2.
11. Wash three times with the abovementioned washing solution.
12. Osmification step, prepare the osmium tetroxide solution inside a fume hood (*see* **Note 5**): 400 μL 0.15% ruthenium red cacodylate solution and 400 μL distilled water, 200 μL 5% aqueous osmium tetroxide solution.
13. Leave samples for 1 h at room temperature.
14. Centrifuge and wash once with 0.1 M cacodylate buffer without ruthenium red.
15. Centrifuge; the final bacterial pellet should look black.

3.4 Embedding in LRWhite Resin of Medium-Grown Bacteria or LRR-Fixed Samples

A common aim of embedding procedures is to obtain morphological information by applying reproducible methods, which can be repeated in any other laboratory as well. Thus, comparable results should be obtained. We have used LRWhite resin with osmification and uranyl acetate treatment as a highly reliable method for embedding various serotypes of pneumococci. Nevertheless, it should be stated that studying, for example, a new clinical isolate of pneumococci with a variety of preparation techniques might result in even better information about the morphological ultrastructure. Especially, when some cryo-based methods like high-pressure freezing and freeze substitution are applied. In common, bacteria are fixed, dehydrated, infiltrated with a liquid resin and after polymerization ultrathin sections of 60–90 nm are cut which are observed under the TEM or in the FESEM applying a STEM detector (for a comprehensive overview *see* [2, 4, 7]).

3.4.1 Fixation and Immobilization in Agar

1. Fixation of the specimen can be routinely performed in the culture medium with final concentrations of 5% formaldehyde (preparation *see* above Subheading 2.3) and 2% glutaraldehyde. Sometimes it is advantageous to perform the formaldehyde fixation at first for 5–15 min than followed by glutardialdehyde fixation. Important: use EM grade glutardialdehyde.

2. Keep the fixed bacteria in the growth medium for at least 1 h at 4–8 °C, then centrifuge and resuspend the pellet in an appropriate buffer. We use routinely cacodylate buffer (0.1 M cacodylate, 0.01 M $CaCl_2$, 0.01 M $MgCl_2$, 0.09 M sucrose, pH 6.9), or alternatively a HEPES buffer (pH 6.9) can be used.
3. Repeat the centrifugation and washing step twice.
4. Resuspend the last pellet in 1% osmium tetroxide either in distilled water or in an appropriate buffer like cacodylate buffer. Perform the osmification at room temperature for 1 h, afterward wash with buffer.

   Important: Always perform osmification in a hood, because osmium tetroxide is very volatile and toxic; always wear eye protection and gloves (*see* **Note 5**).
5. Resuspend the pellet in equal amounts of 2% aqueous agar, which is kept at 45 °C, soak the mixture in a glass Pasteur pipette, and pour the content after a short partial solidification of the agar mixture on a glass slide. Put the glass slide on ice to aid further solidification of the agar. Beginning with this step the LRR-fixed samples are treated as the other samples.
6. After solidification of the agar cut small pieces of 2–3 mm and transfer in a 1.5 or 2.0 mL safe lock tube. This step allows for handling of the samples without performing a centrifugation after every preparation step, so that the dehydration fluid and resin are replaced by soaking and refilling the 1.5/2.0 mL tube.

3.4.2 Dehydration

The aim of this preparation step is to replace preferably all the water in the sample with a fluid, which is miscible both with water and with the embedding resin monomers. Usually ethanol, methanol, and acetone are applied for dehydration. For LRWhite resin ethanol is used. The duration of each dehydration step is kept as short as possible to prevent extraction of components, especially lipids, resulting in subsequent shrinkage of the sample. This is carried out on ice to prevent more pronounced extraction processes.

1. Add the graded series of ethanol (10, 30, and 50%) to a 1.5 mL tube with the specimen and allow it to incubate for 20–30 min for each step on ice depending on the size of the sample.
2. Fill the 1.5 mL tube with 2% uranyl acetate in 70% ethanol and leave overnight at 4–7 °C.
3. Continue the dehydration with 90% and 100% acetone steps on ice.
4. Repeat the 100% acetone step twice on ice.

3.4.3 Embedding with LRWhite Resin

Embedding resin polymers should be soluble in acetone, but for LRWhite dehydration has to be performed in ethanol. The resin should show a low viscosity for better penetration into the sample during infiltration with the resin. In addition, it should polymerize and harden uniformly, thereby producing a sample block hard enough yet plastic enough to be cut into ultrathin sections. Last but not least, it should be stable under electron irradiation in the TEM. None of the available embedding resins fulfil all these characteristics. In our hands, LRWhite resin is preferable to all other embedding resins for embedding of pneumococci (*see* **Note 4**).

1. Infiltrate with LRWhite resin on ice following the scheme: 1 part/volume ethanol: 1 part/volume LRWhite resin for at least 12 h, 1 part/volume ethanol: 2 parts/volumes LRWhite resin for at least 12 h.
2. Pure LRWhite resin without accelerator for 12 h with 2 changes of resin.
3. Pure LRWhite resin with accelerator (1 μL accelerator for 10 mL LRWhite resin.
4. Transfer the specimen to the bottom of a gelatin drug capsule (0.5 mL) and fill the capsule with pure resin.
5. Before sealing the gelatin capsules with the lid place a small notice in the upper part of the capsule written on paper with a pencil to describe the sample. This notice will be polymerized together with the sample.
6. Polymerize the specimen for 2 days at 50 °C with closed gelatin capsules.

3.4.4 Preparing of Ultrathin Sections and Poststaining

Ultrathin sections of specimen should be between 60 and 90 nm thick to allow for proper imaging under a conventional TEM with 80 kV acceleration voltage. Therefore, specimens embedded in gelatin capsules have to be trimmed to obtain a small flat-topped pyramid-like geometry with an area of 0.2–1.0 mm^2. Ultrathin sections are cut using a diamond knife or a glass knife. Since several different types of ultramicrotomes of different companies are on the market the following scheme describes only the main steps in obtaining ultrathin sections (Fig. 4) (*see* **Notes 6** and 7).

1. Trim the specimen with a new razor-blade or a rotating milling cutter with a diamond cutter. The area of the flat-topped pyramid-like structure should be between 0.2 and 1.0 mm^2.
2. Mount the trimmed specimen in the specimen holder of the ultramicrotome, check that the specimen is held firmly by the holder.
3. Insert the specimen holder in the ultramicrotome.
4. Insert the knife with a clearance angle of 4–6° depending on the used knife.
5. Position the specimen parallel to the knife edge.

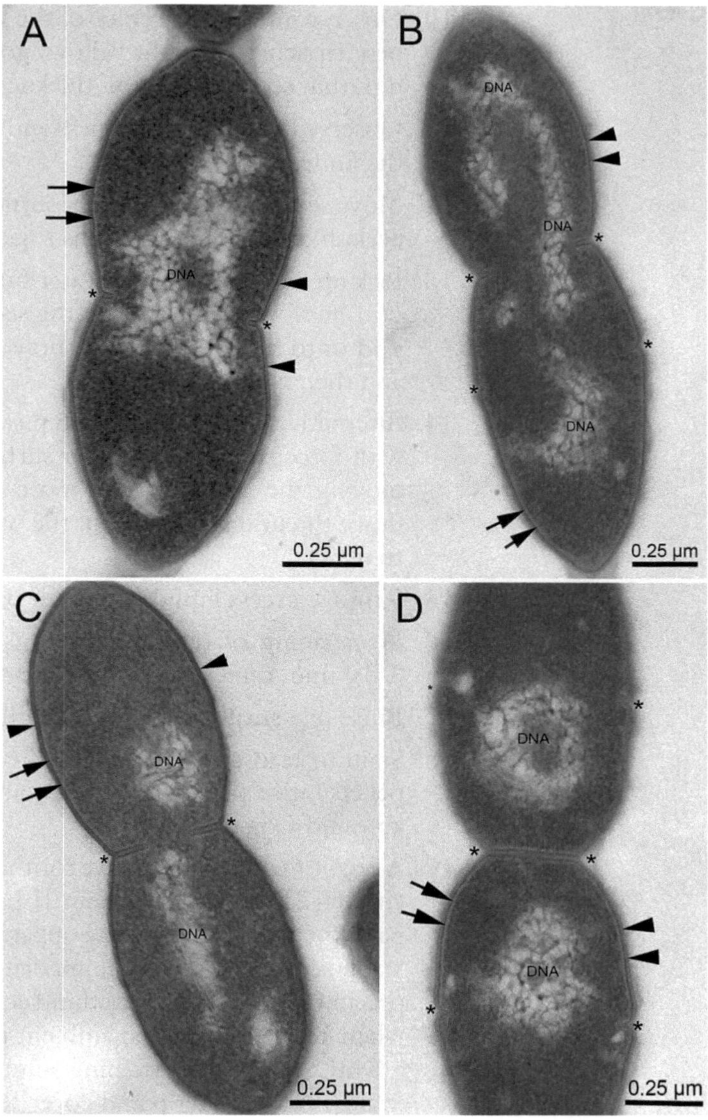

Fig. 4 Series of cell division events of *Streptococcus pneumoniae* TIGR4. (**A–D**) Conventional embedding with aldehyde fixation (5% formaldehyde and 2% glutardialdehyde) in the growth medium, osmification with 1% osmium tetroxide, dehydration with ethanol and embedding in LRWhite hard. Note the overall good preservation of ultrastructural details like cell wall (arrowheads), cytoplasmic membrane (arrows), DNA region, and the different division zones (stars). In addition, cytoplasm shows a high contrast with ribosomes

6. Approach the specimen to the knife edge.
7. Fill the trough with distilled water.
8. Perform 1–3 thick sections of 0.5–1.0 μm.
9. Start cutting with a section thickness of 150 nm.

10. Observe interference color of the section. Adjust section thickness to achieve a light yellow/gold interference color of the ultrathin sections, section thickness is around 60–90 nm.
11. Observe the section thickness and floating of the sections from the knife edge.
12. Move sections onto the water surface with the aid of a mounted eyelash; arrange 2–3 sections together.
13. Pick up sections from the water surface with a Formvar/Butvar grid by slowly approaching the sections from above, press the grid onto sections, allow sections to attach for a few seconds, and then withdraw the grid.
14. Alternatively, sections can be picked up by inserting the grid with forceps under the water surface in the trough and slowly moving the grid upward toward the sections at a 45°. Then move the grid slowly out of the water and sections will adhere to it.
15. Remove excess liquid with filter paper and air-dry.
16. Poststaining of ultrathin sections with 4% uranyl acetate for 3–10 min, omit direct sunlight or illumination (*see* **Note 7**).
17. Rinse in a small beaker with distilled water.
18. Stain in lead citrate in a CO_2-free atmosphere (place NaOH pellets into a petri dish for CO_2 absorption) for 10–30 s (Venable and Goggeshall, 23).
19. A recommended alternative for the Venable & Goggeshall lead citrate [21] is the Ultrostain II package from the Leica company for their grid staining apparatus, since this lead citrate is stabilized, can be used immediately, causes only very minor precipitation on the ultrathin sections and is stable for years when kept in the dark at ambient temperature. For easy use fill a 5 mL syringe with staining solution from the stock solution. Seal with a yellow tip and cover the end of the tip with Parafilm™ to prevent CO_2 influx into the syringe.
20. Rinse the inside the petri dish with drops of boiled distilled water.
21. Rinse with boiled water in a beaker.
22. Air-dry and examine by TEM.
23. Depending if a high or lower contrast is desired on the ultrathin sections it is recommended to start poststaining with uranyl acetate alone and judge the contrast in the TEM before lead citrate staining (*see* **Note 7**).

3.5 Field Emission Scanning Electron Microscopy (FESEM)

3.5.1 Preparation Steps for FESEM

Fixation

Chemical fixation is performed with a fixation solution containing 1–5% formaldehyde (prepared from paraformaldehyde, *see* above Subheading 2.3) and 1–3% glutardialdehyde to preserve the native ultrastructural features. It is recommended to fix the specimen in the growth culture media thus avoiding centrifugation and resuspending of bacteria in a buffer, which might have a detrimental effect on the morphology of the specimen due to too high *g*-forces, especially pneumococci are very sensitive to a harsh treatment.

1. Fixation of the specimen is performed in the culture medium with 5% formaldehyde and 2% glutardialdehyde as end concentration. It is important to use EM grade glutardialdehyde and self-made formaldehyde.
2. Incubate the specimen for at least 1 h at 4–8 °C, centrifuge and resuspend the pellet in TE-buffer, repeat the centrifugation and washing step with TE-buffer. The washing step with TE-buffer reduces the formation of salt crystals on the specimen.

Support for Bacteria in FESEM

Since bacteria represent very tiny specimen they require a support to be imaged in FESEM. Different types of filters (paper filter, nucleopore filter) can be used as a support. But, due to the irregular structures of filters they might mask some morphological features of the specimen when imaged in the FESEM or the structural components are not easily feasible due to the superimposed structures of the support material. Nucleopore filters are better in this respect since they provide a "clean" background but still the numerous pores are visible in the background of the images. For these reasons, our lab established poly-L-lysine-coated 12 mm coverslips as a support for FESEM studies, providing a clean background around the specimen.

1. Add a drop (50 μL) of 0.1% aqueous poly-L-lysine solution on a coverslip and leave for 10 min.
2. Wash the coverslip with distilled water and air-dry.
3. Pipet 50 μL of the fixed and TE-buffer washed specimen solution onto the coverslip. If a lower cell density of bacteria should be examined, dilute the fixed specimen solution with TE-buffer.
4. Allow the fixed specimen solution to stand for 10 min (depending on the size of the bacteria and the number in the solution); thereby, samples can absorb to the poly-L-lysine layer.
5. Transfer the coverslip into a fixation solution of 1% glutardialdehyde in TE-buffer, allow it to stand for 10 min at room temperature, and subsequently wash with TE-buffer.
6. Important: be especially careful not to air-dry your specimen at any step during these preparation steps.

Dehydration

For dehydration a graded series of acetone or ethanol is applied. It is recommended to dry acetone either with $CaCl_2$ or using a molecular sieve before use. The 100% acetone step can also be performed with acetone containing 0.5% water and as a last step with acetone containing only 0.2% water. Ethanol should be used from a freshly opened bottle (*see* **Notes 8–10**).

1. Transfer the coverslip in a small glass petri dish or alternatively into a plastic cell culture plate on ice (depending on the number of coverslips, a 4-well or 24-well plate can be used).
2. Add the graded series of acetone or ethanol (10, 30, 50, 70, and 90%) and allow it to stand for 10–15 min on ice. When changing the solutions, do not pipet the solutions directly on the coverslip; instead, pour it slowly down the plastic wall of the well.
3. Transfer in 100% acetone or ethanol at room temperature in a glass petri dish.
4. Leave for 15 min, replace with new 100% acetone or ethanol and leave it for another 15 min.

Critical Point-Drying

The critical-point drying step has to be performed to obtain a very well prepared specimen for high resolution imaging. For this step in the preparation protocol a critical-point drying (CPD) apparatus is a prerequisite. In principle the specimens, which are prepared in dehydration medium consisting of 100% acetone or ethanol, are transferred into a pressure chamber filled with 100% acetone or ethanol at 8 °C. The chamber is set under pressure and liquid CO_2 is used as a transitional medium. In several exchanges acetone is replace with liquid CO_2. Transition of the liquid CO_2 to gaseous CO_2 is done at the critical pressure for CO_2 (73.8 bar) and the critical temperature at 31 °C. Above the critical point the densities of the drying medium in its liquid and gaseous phases are identical. Therefore, a phase boundary no longer exists. If the temperature is kept above the critical point the gas phase can be slowly vented of the apparatus by a needle valve and the specimen are dried without causing any surface tensions. Since several different CPD apparatus exist, no detailed protocol can be provided. Please refer to the manufacturer's instructions for a given CPD apparatus.

Alternatively, if no CPD apparatus is available a chemical drying procedure with hexamethyldisilazane (HMDS) or tetramethylsilane (TMS) can be applied. This methods works well especially for gram-positive bacteria and some gram-negative bacteria, also for cell cultured cells, but for delicate organisms like Archaea or unknown species it is not recommended.

1. Fixation is the same as for CPD but dehydration of the specimen has to be performed in ethanol.

2. Once the specimen is in 100% ethanol, it must be transferred to 100% HMDS or TMS in a graded series of ethanol-HMDS or TMS mixtures, just cover the specimen with the liquid, perform the infiltration with HMDS or TMS at room temperature.
3. 1 part/volume:1 part/volume, 100% ethanol:100% HMDS or TMS for 10 min.
4. 1 part/volume:2 parts/volumes, 100% ethanol:100% HMDS or TMS for 10 min.
5. 1 part/volume:3 parts/volumes, 100% ethanol:100% HMDS or TMS for 10 min.
6. 1 part/volume:4 parts/volumes, 100% ethanol:100% HMDS or TMS for 10 min, keep in mind that incomplete transition from ethanol into HMDS is a bad source of problems.
7. 100% HMDS or TMS with two changes for 5 min each step; be very cautious that the specimen is not yet air-dried at any time.
8. Exchange once again with 100% HMDS or TMS.
9. Let the specimen completely air-dry, depending on the sample size this takes 10–30 min.

Mounting the Specimen

Due to the hydrophilic character of most biological specimens they should be mounted and sputter-coated immediately. For mounting circles of adhesive tape fitting the size of the sample stub is commonly used and works very well for coverslips.

Sputter Coating of the Specimen

In general, biological specimens are poor electrical conductors. Thus, the sample is prone to charging effects, which might lead to the fact that no imaging at all is possible. Therefore, conductivity must be achieved by coating the specimen with conductive material to perform imaging in a FESEM or other SEMs. In most cases, specimens are sputter-coated with a thin layer of gold (around 5–10 nm, depending on the specimen), because gold is a very good secondary electron emitter. Our laboratory uses routinely gold–palladium. For the detailed protocol please refer to the manufacturer's instructions for the coating apparatus (*see* **Note 11**).

3.6 Cryo-Field Emission Scanning Electron Microscopy (Cryo-FESEM)

When LRR-fixed samples of pneumococcal capsules were imaged in a FESEM after following the conventional preparation protocol as outlined above, the CPS is still aggregating and collapsing due to dehydration steps and critical point-drying [13]. To prevent collapsing of the capsule cryo methods can be applied. In this technology the water in the sample is vitrified without the formation of any ice crystals. It should be mentioned that these cryo methods are mostly time-consuming studies and cannot be performed in a normal electron microscopic laboratory on a regular basis. A detailed preparation protocol depends on the installed cryo system

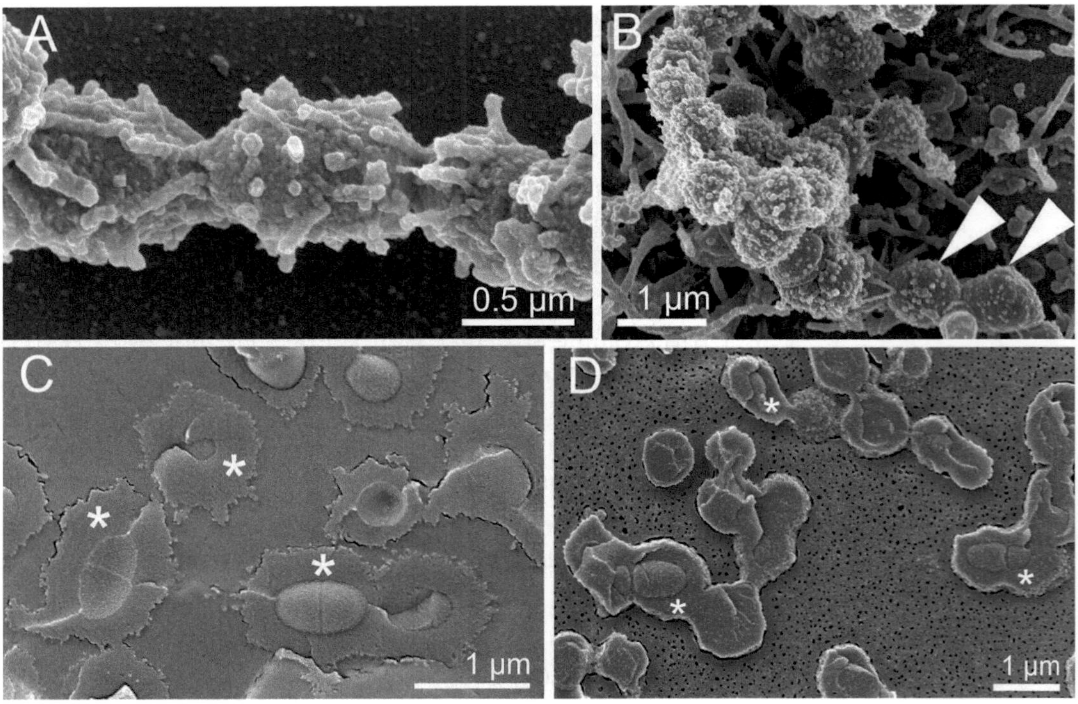

Fig. 5 Cryo field emission scanning microscopy of LRR-fixed pneumococci. (**A**) After LRR fixation and dehydration with acetone FESEM reveals capsular material on the pneumococcal surface. (**B**) After performing an infection on epithelial cells, it was demonstrated that pneumococci being in direct contact with the epithelial cell membrane lose their capsule on contact with the host cell, see arrowheads. Therefore, conventional FESEM was not able to restore the full size of the capsule like in the ultrathin sections. (**C**) and (**D**) In contrast to conventional FESEM, cryo-FESEM allowed for detecting the full size of the pneumococcal capsular polysaccharide after LRR fixation, after normal freeze-etching and deep-freeze etching, stars in (**C**) and (**B**)

on the FESEM. Here we describe the main steps for a cryo preparation (Fig. 5).

1. Centrifuge the LRR-fixed pneumococci.
2. With a needle scratch material of the pellet and fill into the carrier of the cryo system installed at the FESEM.
3. Fill liquid nitrogen in a suitable apparatus and evaporate gas with a pump until nitrogen is solid.
4. Release the light vacuum in the apparatus and bring the carrier with the sample immediately into the melting nitrogen. The sample will be frozen without Leidenfrost's phenomenon.
5. Bring the frozen carrier under nitrogen into the cryo system.
6. With the help of a scalpel fracture the frozen sample.
7. Leave the sample for a given time for etching the fractured surface.

8. Stop etching by sputter coating with gold or gold–palladium (*see* **Note 11**).
9. Insert the carrier into the precooled cryo-stage of the FESEM.
10. Image the sample at the recommended temperature and at a low acceleration voltage like 1–3 kV.
11. For the Gatan HP 1500 system the settings are as follows: freeze-fracture at −105 °C, freeze-etching for 30 s at −105 °C, freeze-etching for deep etching for 2 min at −105 °C, sputter-coating at −105 °C, imaging at −140 °C.

4 Notes

1. For negative staining a concentration of 0.5–1% of aqueous uranyl acetate is recommended for bacteria and 2–4% for proteins and phages.
2. Never use purchased formaldehyde since it contains 10% methanol as a stabilizing agent for preventing polymerization of formaldehyde.
3. Instead of cacodylate buffer which contains barbiturate, HEPES buffer (0.1 M HEPES, 0.09 M sucrose, 0.01 M $MgCl_2$, 0.01 M $CaCl_2$, pH 6.9) can be used.
4. For LRWhite embedding, be aware that opened and older bottles of LRWhite have the tendency to polymerize at lower temperatures than the recommended 50 °C. Even at 25 °C it can start to polymerize partially. Therefore, add the accelerator only at the last step of the infiltration scheme for the resin and keep the sample under 20 °C.
5. Always perform osmification in a hood, because osmium tetroxide is very volatile and toxic, always wear eye protection and gloves (*see* **Note 7**).
6. If ultrathin sectioning of LRWhite samples is not satisfactory, it is recommended to polymerize the trimmed sample for another 12–24 h at 50 °C.
7. For poststaining it is recommended to post-stain first with uranyl acetate alone before applying a double staining with uranyl acetate and lead citrate. The time for lead citrate staining has to be customized for the given sample, that is, start with 10 s and observe the contrast.
8. If dehydration is performed with acetone in a plastic culture plate transfer the coverslips from the 90% acetone step into a glass petri dish because 100% acetone will dissolve the plastic petri dish or directly transfer into the critical point drying holder for the last step of acetone dehydration (*see* **Note 5**).

9. Be extremely careful not to air-dry the specimen at the 100% acetone step during manipulation of the coverslips, since in a warm environment acetone will evaporate rapidly from the specimen. Thus, leaving partially air-dried samples, which exhibit extreme characteristics of surface tension like disrupted eukaryotic cells, membranes with numerous holes and cuts or destroyed bacteria.
10. If dehydration is performed with HMDS or TMS take precautions not to air-dry samples during handling. Air-drying is more pronounced when compared to acetone dehydration.
11. For sputter-coating it is recommended to use gold–palladium (80:20 w/w) because samples can be imaged even after several months without a significant loss in performance when kept in a sealed container at room temperature.

References

1. Armbruster BL, Carlemalm E, Chiovetti R, Garavito LRM, Hobot JA, Kellenberger E, Villinger W (1982) Specimen preparation for electron microscopy using low temperature embedding resin. J Microsc 126:77–85
2. Bozzola JJ, Russel LD (1999) Electron microscopy. Principles and techniques, 2nd edn. Jones and Bartlett, Boston
3. Carlemalm E, Garavito RM, Villiger W (1982) Resin development for electron microscopy and an analysis of embedding at low temperature. J Microsc 126:123–143
4. Glauert AM, Lewis PR (2000) Biological specimen preparation for transmission electron microscopy. In: Glauert AM (ed) Practical methods in electron microscopy, vol 17. Portland Press, London
5. Graham LL, Beveridge TJ (1990) Evaluation of freeze-substitution and conventional embedding protocols for routine electron microscopic processing of eubacteria. J Bacteriol 171:2141–2149
6. Hoppert M (2003) Microscopic techniques in biotechnology. Wiley-VCH, Weinheim
7. Hoppert M, Holzenburg A (1998) Electron microscopy in microbiology. BIOS Scientific Publishers, Oxford
8. Baumeister W, Grimm R, Walz J (1999) Electron tomography of molecules and cells. Trends Cell Biol 9:81–85
9. Springer EL, Roth IL (1973) The ultrastructure of the capsules of *Diplococcus pneumonia* and *Klebsiella pneumonia* stained with ruthenium red. J Gen Microbiol 74:21–31
10. Geno KA, Gilbert GL, Song JY, Skovsted IC, Klugman KP, Jones C, Konradsen HB, Nahm MH (2015) Pneumococcal capsules and their types: past, present, and future. Clin Microbiol Rev 28:871–899
11. Geno KA, Saad JS, Nahm MH (2017) Discovery of novel pneumococcal serotype 35D, a natural WciG-deficient variant of serotype 35B. J Clin Microbiol 55:1416–1425
12. Eberhardt A, Hoyland CN, Vollmer D, Bisle S, Cleverley RM, Johnsborg O, Håvarstein LS, Lewis RJ, Vollmer W (2012) Attachment of capsular polysaccharide to the cell wall in *Streptococcus pneumoniae*. Microb Drug Resist 18 (3):240–255
13. Hammerschmidt S, Wolff S, Hocke A, Rosseau S, Müller E, Rohde M (2005) Illustration of pneumococcal polysaccharide capsule during adherence and invasion of epithelial cells. Infect Immun 73:4653–4667
14. Kim JO, Weiser JN (1998) Association of intrastrain phase variation in quantity of capsular polysaccharide and teichoic acid with the virulence of *Streptococcus pneumoniae*. J Infect Dis 177(2):368–377
15. Fassel TA, Mozdziak PE, Sanger JR, Edmiston CE Jr (1997) Paraformaldehyde effect on ruthenium red and lysine preservation and staining of the staphylococcal glycocalyx. Microsc Res Tech 36:422–427
16. Fassel TA, Mozdziak PE, Sanger JR, Edmiston CE Jr (1998) Superior preservation of the staphylococcal glycocalyx with aldehyde-ruthenium red and select lysine salts using extended fixation times. Microsc Res Tech 41:291–297
17. Fassel TA, Edmiston CE Jr (1999) Ruthenium red and the bacterial glycocalyx. Rev Biotechnol Histochem 74:194–212
18. Luft JH (1971) Ruthenium red and violet. 1. Chemistry, purification, methods of use for

electron microscopy and mechanism of action. Anat Rec 171:347–368

19. Luft JH (1971) Ruthenium red and violet. II. Fine structural localization in animal tissue. Anat Rec 171:369–415

20. Valentine RC, Shapiro BM, Stadtman ER (1968) Regulation of glutamine synthetase. XII. Electron microscopy of the enzyme from *Escherichia coli*. Biochemistry 7:2143–2152

21. Venable JH, Coggeshall R (1965) A simplified lead citrate stain for use in electron microscopy. J Cell Biol 25:407–408

22. Bradley DE (1954) Evaporated carbon films for use in electron microscopy. Br J Appl Phys 5:65–66

Chapter 3

Immunofluorescent Staining and High-Resolution Microscopy to Study the Pneumococcal Cell

Federico Iovino and Birgitta Henriques-Normark

Abstract

Immunofluorescent staining using antibodies to detect specific proteins allows for visualization of proteins of interest in a biological sample. In recent years, there have been important advances in the microscopy equipment used for imaging, and we can now perform so-called high-resolution microscopy. Through high-resolution microscopy we can not only study biological processes but also visualize them.

Key words High-resolution microscopy, Pneumococcal cell, Immunofluorescence

1 Introduction

In order to perform an immunofluorescent staining of a bacterial sample, it is important to start with a new fresh culture of pneumococci. The bacterial growth can either be stopped in exponential phase or stationary phase, preferably before pneumococci start lysing. Immunofluorescent staining of pneumococci can be performed in Eppendorf tubes to make the procedure more practical. An optimal volume of a bacterial culture to start the immunofluorescent staining with is in the range of 200–500 μl. Since during the staining procedure there are several washing steps that eliminate some bacteria, it is wise to start with a sufficient number of bacteria in order to have enough bacteria left for imaging. For correct interpretation of the results it is absolutely crucial to have a consistent number of bacteria.

2 Materials

2.1 Preparation of Antibody Solutions

1. Immunofluorescent detection is performed using antibody solutions diluted in sterile 1× phosphate-buffered saline (PBS) with either 5% fetal calf serum (FCS) or 1% bovine

Federico Iovino (ed.), *Streptococcus pneumoniae: Methods and Protocols*, Methods in Molecular Biology, vol. 1968, https://doi.org/10.1007/978-1-4939-9199-0_3,

serum albumin (BSA) (*see* **Note 1**). To prepare 1 l of 1× PBS, start with 800 ml of distilled water and add 8 g of NaCl, 0.2 g of KCl, 1.44 g of Na_2HPO_4, 0.24 g of KH_2PO_4, adjust the pH to 7.4 with HCl, and finally add distilled water to a total volume of 1 l.

2. To stain pneumococci, if bacteria are encapsulated use anti-capsule antibodies (sera) from Statens Serum Institut (Copenhagen, Denmark) as pneumococcal markers, diluted 1:100 [1, 2]. These capsular antisera are serotype-specific. If primary antibodies specific for certain proteins are used, the dilutions to be used are usually the ones recommended by the manufacturer if the antibody is commercially available. Otherwise a titration of antibody (from 1:50 to 1:200 dilution) is highly recommended in order to determine the optimal antibody dilution to use.
3. Fluorophore-conjugated antibodies are normally used as secondary antibodies for immunofluorescent detection. Dilution of secondary antibodies should range from 1:500 to 1:1000. As mentioned above for the primary antibody, a titration of the secondary antibody should also be performed to determine the optimal antibody dilution to use during the staining procedure.
4. If pneumococci are stained for two antigens simultaneously and the two primary antibodies are raised in two different hosts, for instance a rabbit and a mouse IgG, then the two primary antibodies can be mixed together in the first incubation. Also the secondary antibodies can be mixed together. For example, an anti-rabbit antibody and an anti-mouse secondary antibody, following the example above, can be mixed. Importantly, the two secondary antibodies must me raised in the same host (e.g., goat) to avoid chances of cross-reaction among the antibodies themselves.
5. When pneumococci are stained for two antigens simultaneously and there might be a risk for cross-link issues with the use of the secondary antibodies, primary antibodies can by directly labeled with fluorophores using the Zenon IgG Labeling kits from Thermo Fisher Scientific [1]. Using these kits, primary antibodies are made fluorescent and the use of secondary antibodies is not necessary.

3 Methods

3.1 Immunofluorescent Staining

1. Before starting the staining procedure it is important to set the temperature of the cold centrifuge at 4 °C and keep the centrifuge cold for the entire time of the staining.

2. Bacteria can be either fixed or not fixed. If the antigens are surface exposed, then fixation is not strictly necessary. On the other hand, if antigens are intracellular, fixation with permeabilizing fixatives is required (*see* **Note 2**).
3. The bacterial culture is centrifuged at 9600 × *g* for 5 min at 4 °C and the supernatant (culture medium used for the bacterial growth) is removed. Then the bacterial pellet is resuspended in 100 μl of PFA 4% for 15 min at 4 °C. Then the fixed bacterial suspension is centrifuged at 9600 × *g* for 5 min at 4 °C, and the supernatant is removed and the fixed bacterial pellet is resuspended in 500 μl PBS (*see* **Note 3**). The bacterial suspension is again centrifuged at 9600 × *g* for 5 min at 4 °C and the supernatant is removed.
4. The bacterial pellet is now ready to start the immunostaining procedure. The pellet is resuspended in 100 μl of primary antibody solution and the incubation with primary antibody shall last for 1 h at 4 °C. If the primary antibody has already been coupled with fluorophore using the Zenon IgG Labeling kit, the incubation must be performed in the dark. After this incubation, the bacterial suspension is centrifuged at 9600 × *g* for 5 min at 4 °C and the supernatant removed. Then the pellet is resuspended with 500 μl of PBS-T (*see* **Note 3**) and this washing procedure is repeated again two times (*see* **Note 3**). The pellet is then resuspended in 100 μl of secondary antibody solution. The incubation with the secondary antibody shall last for 1 h at 4 °C. After this incubation, as performed after the incubation with the primary antibody (*see* above), the bacterial suspension is centrifuged at 9600 × *g* for 5 min at 4 °C and the supernatant removed. Then the pellet is resuspended with 500 μl of PBS-T. This washing procedure is repeated three times, twice using 500 μl of PBS-T, and once (the last washing step) using 500 μl of PBS (to remove the Tween).
5. After the final wash in PBS, the pellet is finally resuspended in 100 μl of distilled water and 10 μl drops are pipetted onto a microscope glass slide (typically 75 by 26 mm and 1 mm thick) and dried. Mounting medium (5–10 μl drop) is finally added to each dried drop, covered with a coverslip (either circle, square or rectangle shape, typical thickness 0.13 to 0.17 mm) and analyzed by fluorescence microscopy.

3.2 High-Resolution Microscopy Imaging

1. Microscopy imaging can be performed using a DV Elite Imaging System (Applied Precision), preferably using a scientific complementary metal-oxide-semiconductor (sCMOS) camera for high-resolution [2].
2. Alternatively, imaging can be performed using a confocal microscopy system, as previously used for immunofluorescent staining of pneumococci [1].

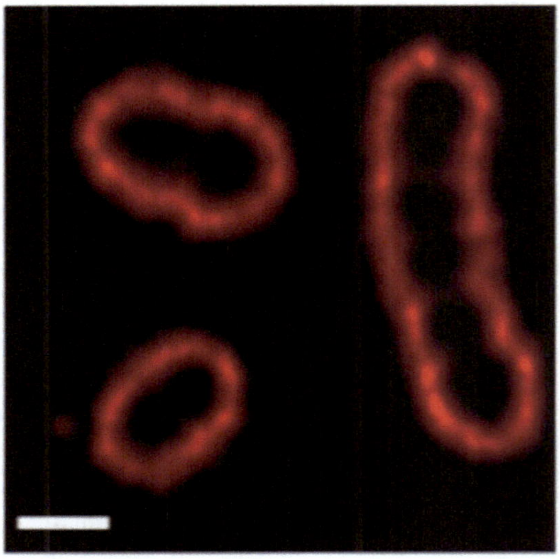

Fig. 1 Immunofluorescent detection of the polysaccharide capsule of *S. pneumoniae*. Immunofluorescent detection of the polysaccharide capsule (blue) of *S. pneumoniae* serotype 6B performed using a specific polyclonal rabbit anti-serotype 6B capsule antibody (primary antibody) in combination with a goat anti-rabbit Alexa Fluor 594 secondary antibody. The scale bar represents 1 μm

3. Images taken with DV Elite Imaging System are acquired using Softworx (Applied Precision) (Fig. 1).
4. Images taken with confocal microscopy systems can be processed using Imaris (Bitplane Scientific Software, Zurich, Switzerland) as previously described [1, 2].

4 Notes

1. FCS and BSA are used to block or at least reduce the nonspecific background staining of the antibody used for the detection of the antigen of interest.
2. Fixation is not always the best; in fact it can damage the protein (s) of interest compromising the intensity and quality of the immunostaining. Especially for antigens exposed on the bacterial cell surface (meaning exposed to the external environment) a staining procedure without fixation can be tried. Immunostaining of pneumococci for detection of capsule or surface-exposed antigens without fixation has been successfully performed and published [3]. If antigens are intracellular, fixation is required and, importantly, in order for antibodies to penetrate inside the bacterial cell, bacterial samples have to be treated with specific fixatives to permeabilize the capsule and the cell wall. Paraformaldehyde (PFA) 4% (prepared in PBS, pH

to be adjusted till reaching the value of 6.9 with HCl solution) is used for fixation. In order to allow antibodies to enter the bacterial cells, the PFA 4% solution is supplemented with 0.1% Triton, a soap used for permeabilization of bacterial cells.

3. Washing steps after fixation and incubation with antibodies are performed, also repeatedly, to remove the excess of fixative or antibodies. If bacterial samples are not properly washed after fixation, traces of fixatives in the bacterial samples can cause disruption of the protein structures leading to possible artifacts in the fluorescent signals. Similarly, washing steps after incubation with antibodies are very important because it is crucial to remove the antibody (either primary or secondary) that has not specifically bound to the antigen of interest. An excess of antibody in the bacterial samples that has not bound specifically can also lead to artifacts such as an excessively bright fluorescent signal. This could happen for instance when an excess of secondary antibody is still present in the bacterial sample. Also, during the last washing step, PBS is used to remove the excess of the soap Tween used in all the previous washing steps.

References

1. Iovino F, Orihuela CJ, Moorlag HE et al (2013) Interactions between blood–borne *Streptococcus pneumoniae* and the blood–brain barrier preceding meningitis. PLoS One 8:e68408
2. Iovino F, Hammarlöf DL, Garriss G et al (2016) Pneumococcal meningitis is promoted by single cocci expressing pilus adhesin RrgA. J Clin Invest 126:2821–2826
3. Iovino F, Molema G, Bijlsma JJ (2014) Platelet endothelial cell adhesion molecule-1, a putative receptor for the adhesion of *Streptococcus pneumoniae* to the vascular endothelium of the blood–brain barrier. Infect Immun 82:3555–3566

Chapter 4

Construction of Fluorescent Pneumococci for In Vivo Imaging and Labeling of the Chromosome

Morten Kjos

Abstract

Advances in fluorescence imaging techniques and development and optimization of fluorescent proteins recent years have made major impacts on different fields of pneumococcal research. This chapter provides methodology for construction of fluorescent pneumococcal strains using fusions to DNA-binding proteins. By expressing fluorescent proteins fused to HlpA, a pneumococcal nucleoid binding protein, brightly fluorescent pneumococci are generated. HlpA fusions may be used both for in vivo imaging of pneumococci as well as for marking the nucleoid in cell biology studies. Furthermore, it also explains how to construct strains for imaging of specific chromosomal loci in pneumococci, using a heterologous ParBS system.

Key words GFP, mKate2, HlpA, Fluorescent fusions, ParB

1 Introduction

Fluorescence microscopy imaging of live cells is instrumental for different fields of pneumococcal research, from mechanistic studies of proteins during various cellular processes to in vivo imaging of bacteria during infection. These techniques rely on the availability of bright fluorescent proteins (FP) and construction of functional protein–FP fusions. Various optimized FPs as well as vectors and methods to construct protein–FP fusions in *Streptococcus pneumoniae* have been described recent years [1–6]. These include FPs of various colors, from green (GFP [4, 6]), red (RFP [1]), yellow (YFP [5]), and cyan (CFP [5]) to FPs optimized for superresolution techniques [7].

In vivo imaging of live pneumococci in infection settings has long been limited by the lack of sufficiently bright FP-expressing cells. In a study from 2015, it was found that FP fusions to the nucleoid binding protein HlpA (SPV_0997, spr1020, histone-like protein A, also referred to as protein HU or Hup) generated bright fluorescent cells suitable for in vivo imaging [8]. Strains expressing HlpA–FP fusions have later been used to image pneumococci

Federico Iovino (ed.), *Streptococcus pneumoniae: Methods and Protocols*, Methods in Molecular Biology, vol. 1968,
https://doi.org/10.1007/978-1-4939-9199-0_4,

during biofilm formation, adherence to epithelial cells, phagocytosis, growth in macrophages, and during infection in a zebrafish meningitis model [8–11]. HlpA–FP fusions have also been utilized as markers for the nucleoid in pneumococcal cell biology studies [1, 3, 6, 12, 13].

While HlpA–FP label the entire nucleoid, other methods are needed to label specific chromosomal loci. One recently developed chromosomal labeling system is based on expression of a heterologous ParB protein (ParB$_P$) derived from the lactococcal plasmid pLP712 (NC_019377). ParB$_P$ binds specifically to an 18-bp palindromic *parS*$_P$ site (GGGGCTAAATTTAGCCCC) [6]. Thus, by simply integrating this 18 bp sequence into the chromosome of strains expressing a ParB$_P$–FP fusion, specific loci of the pneumococcal chromosome can be labeled and visualized by fluorescence microscopy [6]. The pneumococcal chromosome also encodes a ParB-*parS* system, which is involved in chromosome segregation [14]. However, the plasmid-derived ParS$_P$-*parS*$_p$ system used for chromosome labeling here does not interfere with the function of the native, pneumococcal ParB-*parS* [6]. In addition to the ParB$_P$-*parS*$_p$ system, other heterologous chromosomal labeling systems have also recently been published for pneumococci, allowing for visualization of multiple loci simultaneously. These include a TetR/*tetO* repressor–operator system [6] as well as the ParB-*parS* system from *Enterococcus faecalis* [13].

In this chapter, a protocol for construction of strains expressing HlpA-mKate2 is described, in which a *hlpA-mKate2* fusion gene (mKate2 is a far-red RFP) is integrated in tandem with the native pneumococcal *hlpA* [8]. Specific notes on how to generally generate efficient and functional fluorescent fusions in pneumococci are also provided. Secondly, construction of strains with the ParB$_P$-*parS*$_p$ chromosome labeling system is described.

2 Materials

1. Genomic DNA and genome sequence of *S. pneumoniae*.
2. Plasmids
   (a) pMK11-01 or pMK11-02; for amplification of *mKate2* (Addgene #99605 or #99606).
   (b) pPEP1 (Addgene #61046).
   (c) pMK17-02 encoding *parB*$_p^{mut}$*-gfp* (Addgene #99604) (*see* **Note 1**).
   (d) pAE03 (Addgene #61044).
3. Reagents for PCR, including Phusion polymerase, buffer, dNTPs, and primers (Table 1).
4. Equipment for agarose gel electrophoresis.

Table 1
Oligo list

Primer	Alternative name	Sequence (5′–3′); restriction site (underlined); reference
A	hlpA-up-F	AACAAGTCAGCCACCTGTAG; [3]
B	hlpA-R-SphI	CGCGCATGCAGACTGATTATTTAACAGCGTC; SphI; [3]
C	hlpA-F-rbs-SphI	CGTGCATGCTGGAGGAATCATTAACATGGCA; SphI; [3]
D	hlpA-up-R-BamHI	CTGCGGATCCTTTAACAGCGTCTTTAAGAGCTTTACCAGC; BamHI; [3]
E	mKate2-link-BamHI	CGATGGATCCGGATCTGGTGGAGAAGCTGCAGCTAAAGGATC[sp] AGAACTTATCAAGGAAAATATGCACATG; BamHI; [3]
F	mKate2-R-EcoRI	GCATGAATTCTTATTAACGGTGTCCCAATTTACTAG; EcoRI; [3]
G	cam-up-F-EcoRI	ACTCGGAATTCGATAAAAATTTAGGAGGCATATC; EcoRI
H	camR-NotI	ACGTGCGGCCGCTTATAAAAGCCAGTCATTAG; NotI; [3]
I	hlpA-down-F-NotI	AGCGCGGCCGCTTAAAAAGCCTATTGTATCAAGCT; NotI; [3]
J	hlpA-down-R	CGTGGCTGACGATAATGAGG; [3]
K	hlpA-up-check	GATTGTAACCGATTCATCTG; [3]
L	hlpA-down-check	GGAATGCTTGGTCAAATCTA; [3]
M	integration 1	CTTGATGAAACCTACATTTG; [24]
N	integration 2	GCTTCCATTAAGGATAGTTC; [24]
O	integration 3	CCGGTCGCTACCATTACCAG; [24]
P	integration 4	TGGTCTTTAATGATAAAGAA; [24]
Q	rbg-up-F	CAGATCTTCAGAACTATGTCCA; [6]
R	rbg-up-R-BamHI	CCCGGGATCCAGCCTATCTTTTACCCTATATAGA; BamHI; [6]
S	insert-ter-1parSp-BamHI	ATGGATCCGGGGCTAAATTTAGCCCCCAACAGCAAAGAATGGCGGA; BamHI; [6]
T	ery-R-NotI	GTCAGCGGCCGCGTAGGCGCTAGGGACCTC; NotI; [6]
U	rbg-down-F-NotI	GTCAGCGGCCGCAAAAGATAGGGTAAAAGGCTATC; NotI; [6]
V	rbg-down-R	GACCACGACCAACCTCATCA; [6]
W	rbg-check-up	ATCAGATAGTACAGAGGGATC; [6]
X	rbg-check-down	GGCTTGGTCTTGAACGGCT; [6]

5. PCR purification kit.
6. High-fidelity restriction enzymes and buffers: SphI, BamHI, EcoRI, NotI.
7. T4 DNA ligase and buffer.

8. Pneumococcal strain and transformation protocol.
9. Todd Hewitt agar plates (Todd Hewitt broth supplemented with 1.5% agar) with 2 μg/mL chloramphenicol.
10. C+Y-medium [15, 16] or other suitable liquid medium.
    (a) C+Y medium contains (total 110 mL): 100 mL PreC, 2.5 mL Adams III, 2.5 mL 10% yeast extract, 1 mL 8% BSA, 1.5 mL 2% sodium pyruvate, 1 mL 20% glucose, 0.5 mL 2 mg/mL uridine, 0.5 mL 2 mg/mL adenosine, 0.1 mL 0.4 mM $MnCl_2$, 0.073 mL 3% glutamine, 0.327 mL 0.3 M sucrose. pH can be adjusted with HCl.
    (b) PreC contains 8.5 g/L K_2HPO_4, 5 g/L casein hydrolysate, 2 g/L sodium acetate, 11.25 mg/L cysteine, 6 mg/mL tryptophan.
    (c) Adams III contains 24 mg/L biotin, 24 mg/L nicotinic acid, 28 mg/L pyridoxine HCl, 96 mg/L calcium pantothenate, 26 mg/L thiamine HCl, 11 mg/L riboflavin, 20 mg/L $FeSO_4{\cdot}7H_2O$, 20 mg/L $CuSO_4{\cdot}5H_2O$, 20 mg/L $ZnSO_4{\cdot}7H_2O$, 8 mg/L $MnCl_2{\cdot}4H_2O$, 20 g/L $MgCl_2{\cdot}6H_2O$, 1,75 g/L L-asparagine, 200 mg/L choline, 0.5 g/L $CaCl_2$.
11. Induction agents ($ZnCl_2$ and $MnCl_2$).
12. Fluorescence microscope.

3 Methods

3.1 Construction of hlpA-mKate2 Strain

The nucleoid binding protein *hlpA* will be fused to *mKate2*, encoding a monomeric red fluorescent protein [1] (*see* **Note 2**). The fusion construct will integrate immediately downstream of the native *hlpA* gene (*see* **Note 3**) and transcription will thus be driven by the highly active *hlpA* promoter [17] (*see* **Note 4**). The construct is designed to encode a domain-breaking linker (*see* **Note 5**), separating *hlpA* and *mKate2* (RGSGSGGEAAAKGTS). A chloramphenicol resistance gene is placed immediately downstream of *hlpA-mKate2* for selection (*see* **Note 6**). A schematic overview of the construct is shown in Fig. 1, including an outline of how the construct is assembled using conventional restriction and ligation (*see* **Note 7**).

1. Design/order primers corresponding to Fig. 1 and Table 1.
2. Amplify the five DNA fragments using the primer combinations and template DNA indicated in Fig. 1. Standard PCR reactions and PCR cycling conditions are used:

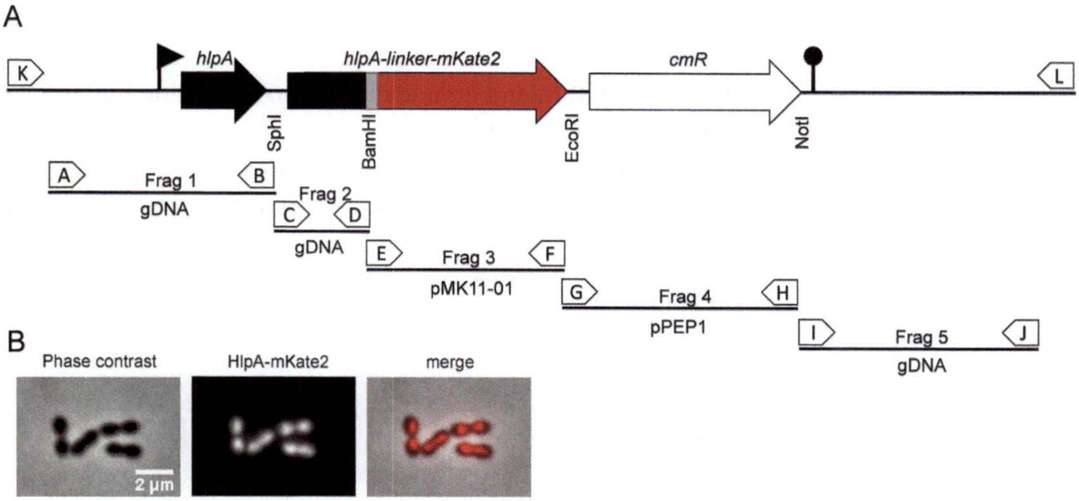

Fig. 1 Construct for expression of HlpA-mKate2. (**a**) Top: Schematic overview of the construction. Flag and lollipop indicate promoter and transcriptional terminator, respectively, while the genes are shown as arrows. Below: Outline of the construction based on amplification of five fragments (Frag 1–5). Restriction sites are indicated and primers are shown as boxed arrows (primers A–L, *see* Table 1). The DNA templates used for amplification are also given. (**b**) Images of *S. pneumoniae* D39 expressing HlpA-mKate2 from the construct above, indicating the nucleoid localized signal. Phase contrast and fluorescence signals are shown individually and merged

Temperature (°C)	Time	
98	5 min	Initial denaturation
98 60 72	20 s 30 s 30 s/kbp	30 cycles
72	10 min	Final elongation

	Volume (μL)
Phusion polymerase	0.5
HF buffer (10×)	10
dNTPs (2.5 mM each)	1
Forward primer (100 μM)	0.5
Reverse primer (100 μM)	0.5
Template DNA (50–100 ng/μL)	1
dH_2O	36.5
Total	50

3. Cast a 1% agarose gel and check that the products are amplified correctly.
4. Purify all PCR fragments and elute in 16 μL elution buffer from the PCR purification kit.
5. Digest fragments 2, 3, and 4 using restriction enzymes BamHI, BamHI/EcoRI, and EcoRI, respectively, using standard reactions.

Component	Volume (μL)
Restriction enzyme	1[a]
Buffer (10×)	2
DNA	16
dH_2O	–[a]
Total	20

[a]1 μL of each restriction enzyme should be used. dH_2O should be added to a total volume of 20 μL.

Incubate the reaction at 37 °C for 30 min.

6. Cast a 1% agarose gel and run the digested fragments on the gel.
7. Purify the digested fragments from gel using a PCR purification kit. Elute in 15 μL from the purification kit.
8. Ligate the fragments. The reaction should be set up with equimolar ratios of the three fragments (1:1:1 molar ratio of each fragment, 1 μL T4 Quick ligase, and 2 μL 10× reaction buffer) at room temperature for 2 h or overnight at 16 °C.
9. Use the ligation mix as template DNA in a PCR reaction (same conditions as above) to amplify the 2 + 3 + 4 fragment using primers C and H.
10. Purify the 2 + 3 + 4 fragment using PCR purification kit.
11. Assemble fragments 1 and 5 to the 2 + 3 + 4 fragment by repeating the procedure in **steps 5–11**; digest fragment 1 with SphI, fragment 2 + 3 + 4 with SphI and NotI and fragment 5 with NotI. Purify the digested fragments and ligate. Finally, amplify the full fragment 1 + 2 + 3 + 4 + 5 using primers A and J.
12. Transform the full linear fragment (Fig. 1) into the *S. pneumoniae* strain. Transformants are selected on TH agar plates containing 2 μg/mL chloramphenicol (*see* **Note 8**).
13. Pick and grow colonies in C+Y medium containing 2 μg/mL chloramphenicol (*see* **Note 9**).
14. Verify transformants by colony PCR using primer pairs K + F and G + L.
15. The resulting strain should display bright fluorescence from the constitutively expressed nucleoid localized fusion protein (Fig. 2).

3.2 Construction of Strain for Localization of Chromosomal Loci Using a Zn^{2+}-Inducible parB$_p$-gfp Fusion

First, a construct for expression of a Zn^{2+}-inducible *parB$_p$^{mut}-gfp* fusion is introduced into the pneumococcal strain.

1. Plasmids encoding fusions of fluorescent proteins to *parB$_p$^{mut}* is available via Addgene (*see* **Note 10**). Transform pMK17-02, encoding *parB$_p$^{mut}-gfp* (*see* **Note 11**) into *S. pneumoniae*. The construct will integrate by double crossover in the *bgaA*-locus of *S. pneumoniae* (*see* **Note 12**). Select transformants on TH agar containing 1 μg/mL tetracycline.
2. Pick colonies and grow in C+Y medium containing 1 μg/mL tetracycline (*see* **Note 9**). Verify integration by colony PCRs using primers M + N and O + P, which will produce a 1 kb product only upon correct integration by double crossover (Fig. 2a).

   Next, a chromosomal locus of choice is tagged by inserting the 18 bp palindromic *parS$_p$* (GGGGCTAAATTTAGCCCC) site into the chromosome. As an example, insertion of *parS$_p$* into the terminus region of the chromosome is explained. The sequence is integrated together with an erythromycin resistance cassette (for selection of transformants) between *rbgA* and *iga* as depicted in Fig. 2.

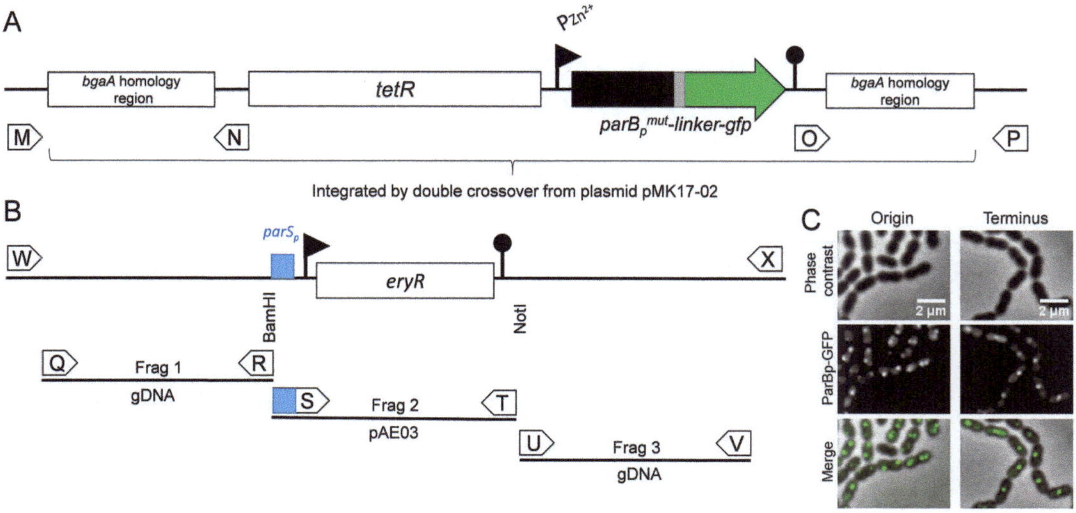

Fig. 2 ParB$_p$-*parS$_p$* chromosome labeling system. **(a)** Schematic overview of the *parB$_p$-gfp* construct integrated in the *bgaA*-locus. **(b)** Schematic overview of the *parS$_p$* integration construct integrated between *rbgA* and *iga* in the terminus region. Promoters are indicated by flags and transcriptional terminators by lollipops. Primers (M-X, *see* Table 1) are shown as boxed arrows and restriction sites are indicated. The 18 bp *parS$_p$* site (GGGGCTAAATTTAGCCCC) is included as overhang in primer S and located upstream of the erythromycin resistance cassette. **(c)** Microscopy images (phase contrast, GFP, and merged images) of pneumococcal strain expressing ParB$_p$-GFP with a *parS$_p$* site introduced close to origin of replication (left panel) or close to the terminus region of the chromosome (right panel)

3. Amplify the three DNA fragments using the primer combinations and template DNA indicated in Fig. 2. Standard PCR reactions and PCR cycling conditions (*see* Subheading 3.1).
4. Purify all PCR fragments.
5. Digest fragments 1, 2, and 3 using restriction enzymes BamHI, BamHI/NotI, and NotI, respectively, using standard reactions (*see* Subheading 3.1).
6. Cast a 1% agarose gel and purify the digested fragments from gel using a PCR purification kit.
7. Ligate the fragments in equimolar ratios (1:1:1 molar ratio of each fragment, 1 μL T4 Quick ligase, and 2 μL 10× reaction buffer) at room temperature for 2 h or overnight at 16 °C.
8. Transform the ligation product directly into the pneumococcal strain made in **step 2**. Select transformants on TH plates containing 0.25 μg/mL erythromycin.
9. Pick and grow transformants in C+Y medium containing 0.25 μg/mL erythromycin (*see* **Note 9**). Verify transformants by PCR using outer primers W + X, and sequence the $parS_p$-site using primer T (Fig. 2).
10. When the strain is verified, it can be used for fluorescence microscopy. To obtain optimal signal strength from the $ParB_p^{mut}$–GFP fusion, first grow the strain in C+Y without antibiotics until OD_{600} = 0.4. Then, dilute the culture 1/100 in C+Y medium. When OD_{600} reach 0.05, add 0.1 mM $ZnCl_2$ and 0.01 mM $MnCl_2$ for induction of $parB_p^{mut}$–*gfp* expression from the Zn^{2+}-promoter. Incubate further until OD_{600} = 0.1–0.2 before performing fluorescence microscopy (*see* **Note 13**).

4 Notes

1. The original $parB_p$-sequence from plasmid pLP712 contains an internal $parS_p$ sequence [6]. This sequence has been mutagenized in $parB_p^{mut}$, which is the version utilized in this protocol.
2. A large number of different fluorescent proteins of various colors have been utilized in protein fusions in pneumococci. Studies have also been performed to compare the performance of different GFP variants [4] and RFP variants [1]. Based on these studies, the GFP of choice is sfGFP(Bs) or its monomeric counterpart m(sf)GFP (Addgene #96603 or #96604), and the RFP of choice is mKate2 (Addgene #96605) for protein–FP fusions. Note, however, that the optimal fluorescent protein will depend on the setup of your fluorescence microscope or fluorescence detection unit, and for superresolution microscopy techniques, fluorescent proteins with specific features are often required.

3. The *hlpA-mKate2* fusion gene is integrated in tandem with the native *hlpA* gene, because introduction of the *hlpA-mKate2* fusion without the presence of a native *hlpA* has not been successful [8]. On the other hand, construction of strains expressing *hlpA* fused to superfolder *gfp* can be made in the absence of a native *hlpA* [8].
4. Expression of *hlpA* fusions has been shown to be highly efficient, producing strains with bright fluorescence [8]. In cases where expression levels of fluorescent fusions are too low, several adjustments can be made for optimization; these include ectopic expression with an inducible promoter (*see* Subheading 3.2) and adding N-terminal tags of 5–10 amino acids to increase translation efficiency [2, 5]. The latter is particularly usable for fusions where the fluorescent protein is fused to the N-terminus of the target protein.
5. To provide structural flexibility between the fluorescent protein and the target proteins, a linker sequence should be added. Different linkers have been utilized in pneumococci [2, 5, 18], including the domain-breaking linker [19] in the *hlpA-mKate2* construct.
6. Other antibiotic resistance genes could be used instead. In this case, the resistance gene is driven by the *hlpA*-promoter. In other cases, it may be necessary to include full resistance cassette (i.e., promoter–resistance gene–terminator) to obtain sufficiently high expression.
7. Any cloning strategy for fusing multiple fragments can in principle be used, including overlap-extension PCR [20], infusion cloning [21, 22], or Gibson (isothermal) assembly [1, 23].
8. Chloramphenicol concentrations ranging from 2 to 4.5 μg/mL can be used for selection, depending on the pneumococcal strain.
9. Instead of picking and growing the colonies in liquid medium containing antibiotics, the colonies can also be replated on antibiotic plates and incubated overnight. Replated colonies can then be picked and grown in liquid medium without antibiotics.
10. In addition to pMK17-02, which is used here, other versions of similar plasmids are available, including pMK17-01 encoding $parB_p$-*gfp* (Addgene #99603), pMK11-01 encoding $parB_p$-*mKate2* (Addgene #99605) pMK11-02 encoding $parB_p^{mut}$-*mKate2* (Addgene #99606).
11. The *gfp* version in this plasmid is monomeric superfolder *gfp*, *m(sf)gfp* [6]. Utilizing monomeric versions is an advantage in many applications to avoid artefacts due to multimerization of the fluorescent proteins.

12. The homology regions to *bgaA* in the plasmid are from the strain D39. Utilization of this plasmid for integration into other pneumococcal strains will depend on the degree of similarity to the sequence of D39, and this should be checked prior to starting the experiment.
13. The best signal is observed when cells are in early and mid-exponential growth phase.

References

1. Beilharz K, van Raaphorst R, Kjos M, Veening JW (2015) Red fluorescent proteins for gene expression and protein localization studies in *Streptococcus pneumoniae* and efficient transformation with DNA assembled via the Gibson assembly method. Appl Environ Microbiol 81:7244–7252
2. Eberhardt A, Wu LJ, Errington J, Vollmer W, Veening JW (2009) Cellular localization of choline-utilization proteins in *Streptococcus pneumoniae* using novel fluorescent reporter systems. Mol Microbiol 74:395–408
3. Kjos M, Veening JW (2014) Tracking of chromosome dynamics in live *Streptococcus pneumoniae* reveals that transcription promotes chromosome segregation. Mol Microbiol 91:1088–1105
4. Overkamp W, Beilharz K, Detert Oude Weme R, Solopova A, Karsens H, Kovacs A, Kok J, Kuipers OP, Veening JW (2013) Benchmarking various green fluorescent protein variants in *Bacillus subtilis*, *Streptococcus pneumoniae*, and *Lactococcus lactis* for live cell imaging. Appl Environ Microbiol 79:6481–6490
5. Henriques MX, Catalao MJ, Figueiredo J, Gomes JP, Filipe SR (2013) Construction of improved tools for protein localization studies in *Streptococcus pneumoniae.* PLoS One 8: e55049
6. van Raaphorst R, Kjos M, Veening JW (2017) Chromosome segregation drives division site selection in *Streptococcus pneumoniae.* Proc Natl Acad Sci U S A 114:E5959–E5968
7. Jacq M, Adam V, Bourgeois D, Moriscot C, Di Guilmi AM, Vernet T, Morlot C (2015) Remodeling of the Z-ring nanostructure during the *Streptococcus pneumoniae* cell cycle revealed by photoactivated localization microscopy. MBio 6:e01108–e01115
8. Kjos M, Aprianto R, Fernandes VE, Andrew PW, van Strijp JA, Nijland R, Veening JW (2015) Bright fluorescent *Streptococcus pneumoniae* for live-cell imaging of host-pathogen interactions. J Bacteriol 197:807–818
9. Ercoli G, Fernandes VE, Chung WY, Wanford JJ, Thomson S, Bayliss CD, Straatman K, Crocker PR, Dennison A, Martinez-Pomares L et al (2018) Intracellular replication of *Streptococcus pneumoniae* inside splenic macrophages serves as a reservoir for septicaemia. Nat Microbiol 3:600–610
10. Jim KK, Engelen-Lee J, van der Sar AM, Bitter W, Brouwer MC, van der Ende A, Veening JW, van de Beek D, Vandenbroucke-Grauls CM (2016) Infection of zebrafish embryos with live fluorescent *Streptococcus pneumoniae* as a real-time pneumococcal meningitis model. J Neuroinflammation 13:188
11. Reddinger RM, Luke-Marshall NR, Sauberan SL, Håkansson AP, Campagnari AA (2018) *Streptococcus pneumoniae* modulates *Staphylococcus aureus* biofilm dispersion and the transition from colonization to invasive disease. MBio 9:e02089–e02017
12. Nourikyan J, Kjos M, Mercy C, Cluzel C, Morlot C, Noirot-Gros MF, Guiral S, Lavergne JP, Veening JW, Grangeasse C (2015) Autophosphorylation of the bacterial tyrosine-kinase CpsD connects capsule synthesis with the cell cycle in *Streptococcus pneumoniae.* PLoS Genet 11:e1005518
13. Mercy C, Lavergne J-P, Slager J, Ducret A, Garcia PS, Noirot-Gros M-F, Dubarry N, Nourikyan J, Veening J-W, Grangeasse C (2018) RocS drives chromosome segregation and nucleoid occlusion in *Streptococcus pneumoniae.* bioRxiv doi: 10.1101/359943
14. Attaiech L, Minnen A, Kjos M, Gruber S, Veening JW (2015) The ParB-*parS* chromosome segregation system modulates competence development in *Streptococcus pneumoniae.* MBio 6:e00662
15. Lacks S, Hotchkiss RD (1960) A study of the genetic material determining an enzyme in pneumococcus. Biochim Biophys Acta 39:508–518
16. Martin B, Garcia P, Castanie MP, Claverys JP (1995) The *recA* gene of *Streptococcus pneumoniae* is part of a competence-induced operon

and controls lysogenic induction. Mol Microbiol 15:367–379

17. Aprianto R, Slager J, Holsappel S, Veening J-W (2018) High-resolution analysis of the pneumococcal transcriptome under a wide range of infection-relevant conditions. Nucleic Acids Res 46:9990-10006
18. Straume D, Stamsås GA, Berg KH, Salehian Z, Håvarstein LS (2017) Identification of pneumococcal proteins that are functionally linked to penicillin-binding protein 2b (PBP2b). Mol Microbiol 103:99–116
19. Arai R, Ueda H, Kitayama A, Kamiya N, Nagamune T (2001) Design of the linkers which effectively separate domains of a bifunctional fusion protein. Protein Eng 14:529–532
20. Higuchi R, Krummel B, Saiki RK (1988) A general method of *in vitro* preparation and specific mutagenesis of DNA fragments: study of protein and DNA interactions. Nucleic Acids Res 16:7351–7367
21. Irwin CR, Farmer A, Willer DO, Evans DH (2012) In-fusion(R) cloning with vaccinia virus DNA polymerase. Methods Mol Biol 890:23–35
22. Liu X, Gallay C, Kjos M, Domenech A, Slager J, van Kessel SP, Knoops K, Sorg RA, Zhang JR, Veening JW (2017) High-throughput CRISPRi phenotyping identifies new essential genes in *Streptococcus pneumoniae*. Mol Syst Biol 13:931
23. Gibson DG (2011) Enzymatic assembly of overlapping DNA fragments. Methods Enzymol 498:349–361
24. Slager J, Kjos M, Attaiech L, Veening JW (2014) Antibiotic-induced replication stress triggers bacterial competence by increasing gene dosage near the origin. Cell 157:395–406

Chapter 5

High-Resolution and Super-Resolution Immunofluorescent Microscopy Ex Vivo to Study Pneumococcal Interactions with the Host

Federico Iovino and Birgitta Henriques-Normark

Abstract

In vivo imaging, meaning imaging tissues in living animals, is still a developing technique. However, microscopy imaging ex vivo remains a very important tool that allows for visualization of biological and pathological processes occurring in vivo. As described in Chap. 5, imaging of animal and human tissue postmortem can be performed at high resolution. Recently, imaging of human tissues infected with pneumococci using an even higher resolution, the so-called super-resolution with STED, has been reported.

Key words High-Resolution microscopy, Super-Resolution, Mouse tissue, Human tissue, Immunofluorescence

1 Introduction

In order to obtain an immunofluorescent staining of a good quality it is important to harvest the organ without damaging the tissues. The storage of the collected organs is crucial for the optimal conservation of the tissue, especially for mid/long-term storages. For immunofluorescent stainings, cryopreservation is recommended; however, it has recently been described that also embedding in paraffin, which is most frequently adopted for immunohistochemistry, can also be used with good results. For cryopreservation, harvested organs are embedded in matrix (cryomatrix) for storage at low temperatures (−80 °C). While for paraffin embedding, tissues are dehydrated through a series of graded ethanol incubation steps to remove the water, and afterward infiltrated with wax. The tissues are then embedded into blocks of wax (paraffin). A very important step for good performance of immunofluorescent stainings is cutting the tissue with a cryostat, for cryopreserved tissues, or with a microtome, for paraffin-embedded tissues. The cutting should be performed in order to have a flat

Federico Iovino (ed.), *Streptococcus pneumoniae: Methods and Protocols*, Methods in Molecular Biology, vol. 1968, https://doi.org/10.1007/978-1-4939-9199-0_5,

surface of the tissue, since a flat tissue surface allows a homogeneous binding of the antibodies, which should provide a uniform fluorescent signal over the whole tissue. In addition, a flat tissue surface is preferred to maintain focus during the microscopy imaging. For imaging of animal and human tissue infected with pneumococci, tissue sections 5 to 30 μm thick have been previously used with good results in immunofluorescent stainings. The thickness is normally decided based on the cell types that are to be detected (*see* **Note 1**).

2 Materials

2.1 Preparation of Antibody Solutions

1. Immunofluorescent detection is performed using antibody solutions diluted in sterile 1× phosphate-buffered saline (PBS) with either 5% fetal calf serum (FCS) or 1% bovine serum albumin (BSA) (*see* **Note 1**). To prepare 1 l of 1× PBS, start with 800 ml of distilled water and add 8 g of NaCl, 0.2 g of KCl, 1.44 g of Na_2HPO_4, 0.24 g of KH_2PO_4, adjust the pH to 7.4 with HCl, and finally add distilled water to a total volume of 1 l.
2. To stain pneumococci, if bacteria are encapsulated use anti-capsular antibodies (sera) from Statens Serum Institut (Copenhagen, Denmark) as pneumococcal markers, diluted 1:100 [1, 2]. Such capsular sera are serotype-specific. If primary antibodies specific for certain proteins are used, the dilutions to be used are usually those recommended by the manufacturer, if the antibody is commercially available. Otherwise a titration of antibodies (from 1:50 to 1:200 dilution) is highly recommended in order to determine the optimal antibody dilution to use.
3. Fluorophore-conjugated antibodies are frequently used as secondary antibodies for immunofluorescent detection. Dilution of secondary antibodies should range from 1:500 to 1:1000, as mentioned above for the primary antibody. A titration of secondary antibodies should be performed to determine the optimal antibody dilution to be used during the staining procedure.
4. To stain cellular nuclei, a DAPI solution is usually used, a recommended range of dilution is 1:2.000 to 1:10.000, the dilution is made in PBS. For host tissue detection, anti-cytokeratin (CK) 8 antibody can be used to detect the lung epithelium, while for the vascular endothelium DyLight 594-labeled *Lycopersicon esculentum*, the so-called tomato lectin (Vector Laboratories), diluted 1:100 (in PBS) can be used [1, 2].

5. To stain specific host proteins, primary antibodies targeting those proteins should be used. The secondary antibodies should be directed to the same host in which the primary antibody has been raised.
6. For STED super-resolution imaging, ATTO secondary antibodies are highly recommended, especially for detection using far-red fluorescent dyes.

3 Methods

3.1 Immuno-fluorescent Staining

1. For pneumococcal infections, ex vivo microscopy imaging is usually performed using lung (in the case of pneumonia) or brain (in the case of meningitis) animal/human tissue sections postmortem [1, 3]. Heart and spleen tissue sections are also used, as it has been recently reported that pneumococci can invade the myocardium and can replicate inside splenic macrophages [4–6]. Cryopreserved or paraffin-embedded tissue sections are cut with a cryostat/microtome and placed on microscope glass slides (three sections/slide is recommended).
2. Sections are fixed with pure acetone for 10 min (*see* **Note 2**), dried and incubated with primary antibody solutions.
3. Usually both pneumococci and host tissue/cells are detected in immunofluorescent stainings ex vivo of animal/human tissue sections. For this reason, tissue sections are incubated with a combination of anti-pneumococcal antibody (to stain the capsule with serotype-specific capsular antibody/sera, or any other specific pneumococcal protein with a specific primary antibody) and a primary antibody specific for the host tissue/cell protein.
4. Before starting the staining procedure, PAP pen is used to create a thin film-like hydrophobic barrier that is drawn around the tissue section. This barrier will allow the antibody solution to remain just on the area of the tissue section without being spread onto the entire surface of the glass slide. Tissue sections are then left at room temperature for a few minutes to allow the PAP pen barriers drawn around them to dry properly.
5. Before starting incubation with antibodies, microscope slides with tissue sections should be wet with PBS to allow a good adherence of the antibody solutions onto the glass slide. Afterward, slides are incubated with primary antibody solution (combination of primary antibodies to stain pneumococci/pneumococcal protein and host cell/tissue). The incubation with primary antibodies shall last for 1 h at room temperature.

6. Slides are then washed twice in PBS, and each incubation in PBS shall last for 5 min (room temperature). It is important to change PBS for every incubation to avoid that slides are washed with PBS that is not clean.
7. Then, slides are incubated with the appropriate secondary antibody solution (combination of secondary antibodies specific for the primary antibodies used in the first incubation). Incubation with the secondary antibodies shall last for 1 h in the dark at room temperature.
8. The slides are then washed in PBS twice, and each incubation in PBS shall last for 5 min (room temperature, dark). If cellular nuclei should be detected as well, DAPI solution is applied on the tissue sections. The incubation with DAPI solution shall last for 10–15 min (room temperature, dark) and slides are washed twice in PBS (each incubation for 5 min, room temperature, dark).
9. After the last washing step, mounting medium is added on each tissue section. Normally drops of 5–10 μl medium are enough for each section and coverslips are applied on each section (*see* **Note 3**). Then slides are ready for microscopy imaging.

3.2 High-Resolution Microscopy Imaging

1. Microscopy imaging can be performed using a DV Elite Imaging System (GE Healthcare), preferably using a scientific complementary metal-oxide-semiconductor (sCMOS) camera for high-resolution [2].
2. Alternatively, imaging can be performed using a confocal microscopy system [1] (Fig. 1).
3. Images taken with DV Elite Imaging System are acquired using Softworx (Applied Precision) (Fig. 1).
4. Images taken with confocal microscopy systems can be processed using Imaris (Bitplane Scientific Software) as previously described [1, 2].

3.3 Super-Resolution Microscopy Imaging

Recently it was shown that super-resolution imaging can be performed of human brain biopsies infected with pneumococci using Stimulated emission depletion (STED) microscopy [3]. According to these recently published results, super-resolution imaging is first performed with a confocal microscopy system with a four-mirror beam scanner, and then with multicolor (two or even three colors) STED imaging. Briefly, the fluorescent signal is collected through the same objective, separated from the excitation path through a dichroic mirror, and then passed through a confocal pinhole. Finally, the resulting signal is then split by a dichroic mirror and detected by two single photon counting detectors that are equipped with separate emission filters and a common infrared (IR)-filter to suppress any scattered light from the STED laser and confer to the image the so-called super-resolution. In fact,

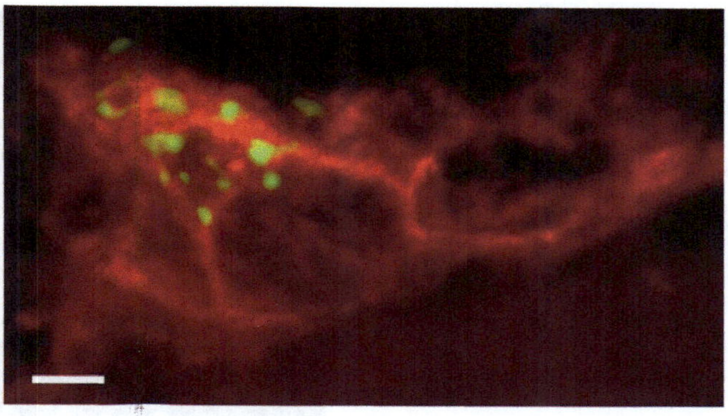

Fig. 1 Immunofluorescent staining of *S. pneumoniae* cells interacting with murine blood–brain barrier detected through high-resolution microscopy imaging. Using brain tissue sections from a mouse systemically infected with *S. pneumoniae*, immunofluorescent detection through high-resolution microscopy showed that serotype 4, strain TIGR4, pneumococci (green), detected with anti-serotype 4 capsule antibody combined with goat anti rabbit Alexa Fluor 488, adhered to the blood–brain barrier endothelium (red) detected with DyLight 594-labeled Lycopersicon Esculentum (tomato lectin). Scale bar represents 5 μm. Imaging was performed with a confocal microscopy system

using this imaging technique, a spatial resolution of about 25 nm can be reached. Image acquisition is controlled using a FPGA-card and processed with the Imspector software (Abberior Instruments) (Fig. 2).

4 Notes

1. The thickness of the tissue section is normally decided based on the size of the cell type/antigens that are detected during the immunostaining. Pneumococcal cells are usually from one to a few micrometers thick, depending on whether the bacteria are in the form of single cocci or chains. If also the host tissue is detected, normally endothelium and epithelium layers can be properly stained and imaged with tissue sections that are a few micrometers thick. Thus, recommended thickness can vary within a range of 5–10 μm. On the other hand, if other cell types are stained, like microglia, neurons, or astrocytes in the brain tissue, then a bigger thickness should be considered [1–3]. Some cells can have a bigger size due to the long cellular processes/dendrites, and then a thickness of 20–30 μm is recommended [1–3].
2. Fixation with acetone confers a better histological preservation of the tissue and conserves epitopes to a high degree. Furthermore, acetone is a permeabilizing fixative which means that after acetone fixation intracellular antigens can be detected.

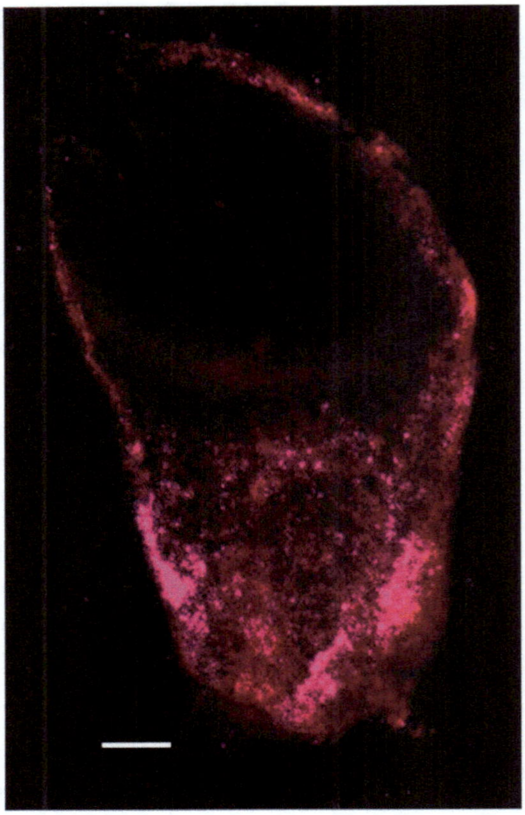

Fig. 2 Immunofluorescent staining of *S. pneumoniae* cells interacting with human blood–brain barrier detected through STED super-resolution microscopy imaging. Using brain biopsies from patients with pneumococcal meningitis, immunofluorescent detection through super-resolution microscopy showed that serotype 19F pneumococci (purple), detected with a rabbit anti-capsule antibody in combination with a goat anti-rabbit ATTO 647 secondary antibody, adhered to the PECAM-1 receptor (red), detected with a rat anti-human PECAM-1 antibody in combination with a goat anti-rat Alexa Fluor 594 secondary antibody, expressed on the blood–brain barrier endothelium (red), detected with DyLight 594-labeled Lycopersicon Esculentum (tomato lectin). Scale bar represents 1 μm. Imaging was performed with a STED super-resolution microscopy system

Concerning the importance of permeabilization of the samples to be stained, *see* **Note 2** of Chap. 3.

3. When coverslips are applied onto the mounting medium, it is important to reduce at minimum the formation of air bubbles on the tissue section. If some air bubbles are formed, which is quite inevitable, it is good to gently press the coverslips onto the glass slide with the tip of a 20–100 μl pipette, trying to push away air bubbles from the tissue sections.

References

1. Iovino F, Hammarlöf DL, Garriss G et al (2016) Pneumococcal meningitis is promoted by single cocci expressing pilus adhesin RrgA. J Clin Invest 126:2821–2826
2. Iovino F, Orihuela CJ, Moorlag HE et al (2013) Interactions between blood-borne *Streptococcus pneumoniae* and the blood–brain barrier preceding meningitis. PLoS One 8:e68408
3. Iovino F, Engelen-Lee JY, Brouwer M et al (2017) pIgR and PECAM-1 bind to pneumococcal RrgA and PspC mediating bacterial invasion of the brain. J Exp Med 214:1619–1630
4. Ercoli G, Fernandes VE, Chung WY et al (2018) Intracellular replication of *Streptococcus pneumoniae* inside splenic macrophages serves as a reservoir for septicaemia. Nat Microbiol 3:600–610
5. Shenoy AT, Brissac T, Gilley RP et al (2017) *Streptococcus pneumoniae* in the heart subvert the host response through biofilm-mediated resident macrophage killing. PLoS Pathog 13:e1006582
6. Brown AO, Mann B, Gao G et al (2014) *Streptococcus pneumoniae* translocates into the myocardium and forms unique microlesions that disrupt cardiac function. PLoS Pathog 10:e1004383

Part III

The Genetics of *Streptococcus pneumoniae*

Chapter 6

Natural Genetic Transformation: A Direct Route to Easy Insertion of Chimeric Genes into the Pneumococcal Chromosome

Isabelle Mortier-Barrière, Nathalie Campo, Mathieu A. Bergé, Marc Prudhomme, and Patrice Polard

Abstract

The ability of *Streptococcus pneumoniae* (the pneumococcus) to transform is particularly convenient for genome engineering. Several protocols relying on sequential positive and negative selection strategies have been described to create directed markerless modifications, including deletions, insertions, or point mutations. Transformation with DNA fragments carrying long flanking homology sequences is also used to generate mutations without selection but it requires high transformability. Here, we present an optimized version of this method. As an example, we construct a strain harboring a translational fusion *ftsZ-mTurquoise* at the *ftsZ* locus. We provide instructions to produce a linear DNA fragment containing the chimeric construction and give details of the conditions to obtain optimal pneumococcal transformation efficiencies.

Key words Natural genetic transformation, Gene transfer, Markerless integration/mutagenesis, Overlapping PCR

1 Introduction

The bacterium *Streptococcus pneumoniae* is particularly accessible to genetic manipulation via the process of natural transformation, which is remarkably efficient in this species. Transformation is a horizontal gene transfer mechanism that facilitates the introduction of multiple types of mutations into the chromosome. Point mutations, deletions and insertions (e.g., fluorescent reporters, affinity tags, and binding sequences) can be introduced into a single starting strain without using selectable markers. Construction of markerless mutants avoids the accumulation of drug resistance genes and other extraneous sequences that may complicate genetic modifications and interfere with gene expression. A common method for creating markerless mutations into the pneumococcal genome is the Janus technique [1], a two-step transformation procedure

Federico Iovino (ed.), *Streptococcus pneumoniae: Methods and Protocols*, Methods in Molecular Biology, vol. 1968, https://doi.org/10.1007/978-1-4939-9199-0_6,

based on sequential positive and negative selection of streptomycin resistance. Although efficient, this approach is time-consuming owing to the numerous constructions needed and is bedeviled by false positives arising from gene conversion. The Cheshire cassette method [2], based on site-specific recombination by Cre at *lox*P sites, appears more straightforward. However, it is largely restricted to generating deletions, and the final excision step leaves a 34 bp *lox*P site at the target site. Another method consists in a single transformation step with a chimeric donor DNA fragment carrying long flanking homology sequences produced by overlap extension PCR. No cloning and no additional enzymatic reaction, such as DNA ligation or DNA digestion, is necessary for generation of these constructs. In 2004, Iannelli and Pozzi [3] presented a detailed protocol for this technique yielding in-frame deletions and insertions at frequencies of about 1%. More recently, Junges and colleagues [4] published an improved version of this method that enables introduction of point mutations into pneumococcal genes with high efficiency. Here, we describe a variant of this protocol that allows the routine generation of unlabeled insertions and deletions of about 1 kb at efficiencies of 10% to 20% and of point mutations at greater than 80%. The efficiency of markerless genome modifications depends on the transformability of the competent cells, the quality and quantity of the donor DNA and the size of homologous regions for integration. To illustrate this method, we present the construction of a strain containing a chimeric translational fusion of the genes encoding the fluorophore mTurquoise2 and the FtsZ protein, which assembles at the division plane of growing cells (Fig. 1). This construction results in the insertion at the *ftsZ* locus of a 720 bp heterologous fragment containing the *mTurquoise2* DNA sequence. We first explain how to design the primers to generate the chimeric fusion. We then list the steps taken to produce a PCR DNA fragment carrying the *ftsZ-mTurquoise* fusion. Finally, we detail the conditions used to obtain optimal frequencies of transformation with synthetic chimeric donor DNA fragments.

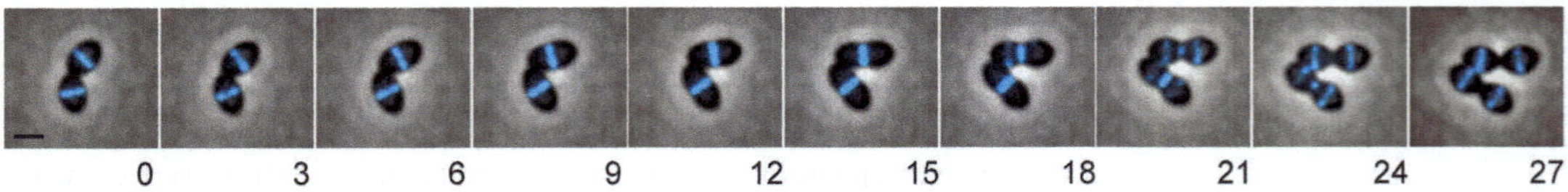

Fig. 1 Strain producing the chimeric translational FtsZ-mTurquoise2 fusion (R4011). Still images from fluorescence time-lapse microscopy of R4011 at 37 °C. Acquisition times in minutes are indicated. Overlays between phase contrast (gray) and mTurquoise (blue) are shown. Scale bar, 1 μm

2 Materials

Prepare all media and solutions using ultrapure water with resistivity of $\leq$18.2 MΩ cm at 25 °C (milliQ-water).

2.1 Growth Media

1. C+Y medium (*see* **Note 1**) composition: casein hydrolysate (5 g L^{-1}), tryptophan (6 mg L^{-1}), cysteine (11.25 mg L^{-1}), CH_3COONa (2 g L^{-1}), K_2HPO_4 (8.5 g L^{-1}), $MgCl_2{\cdot}6H_20$ (0.5 g L^{-1}), $CaCl_2$ (12.5 mg L^{-1}), $MnCl_2$ (250 μg L^{-1}), $FeSO_4{\cdot}7H_2O$ (0.5 mg L^{-1}), $CuSO_4{\cdot}5H_2O$ (0.5 mg L^{-1}), $ZnSO_4{\cdot}7H_2O$ (0.5 mg L^{-1}), biotin (0.6 μg L^{-1}), nicotinic acid (0.6 mg L^{-1}), pyridoxine hydrochloride (0.7 mg L^{-1}), thiamine hydrochloride (0.6 mg L^{-1}), riboflavin (0.3 mg L^{-1}), calcium pantothenate (2.4 mg L^{-1}), L-asparagine·H_2O (50 mg L^{-1}), uridine (20 mg L^{-1}), adenosine (20 mg L^{-1}), glutamine (22 mg L^{-1}), sodium pyruvate (0.3 g L^{-1}), sucrose (0.3 g L^{-1}), glucose (2 g L^{-1}), bovine serum albumin (0.8 g L^{-1}), choline (5 mg L^{-1}), and yeast extract (25 g L^{-1}) [5]. The preparation recipe is detailed in **Note 2**.
2. CAT-agar medium composition: dextrose (1 g L^{-1}), sodium chloride, NaCl (5 g L^{-1}), Trizma base (1.25 g L^{-1}), yeast extract (1 g L^{-1}), Bacto tryptone (5 g L^{-1}), Bacto Casitone (10 g L^{-1}), and agar (10 g L^{-1}).
3. THY medium composition: Bacto Todd Hewitt (30 g L^{-1}), yeast extract (5 g L^{-1}).

2.2 Strains

1. R304: *str41, rif23, nov1;* SmR, RifR, NovR [6].
2. R1502: *comC0, ssbB::*pR424 (*luc*); CmR [7].
3. R4011: *comC0, ssbB::*pR424 (*luc*), *ftsZ-mTurquoise*; CmR (this study).

2.3 Antibiotic

Streptomycin: 200 mg mL^{-1} stock; concentration in medium 200 μg mL^{-1}.

2.4 Kit

Illustra GFX™ DNA and Gel Band Purification Kit—GE Healthcare.

2.5 Primers

Primers are listed in Table 1.

Table 1
Primers used in this study

Name	Sequences (nt)
oIM90 forward	GCTACAGTGATTGATATGGGGGCAGG (26 nt)
oIM67[a] reverse	**CAATTCTTCACCTTTAGAAACCAT**TCCGGAACCCTCGAG*ACGATTTTTGAAAA [sp] ATGGAGGTGTATCC* (67 nt)
oIM68[a] forward	*GGATACACCTCCAT[sp] TTTTCAAAAATCGT*CTCGAGGGTTCCGGA[sp] **ATGGTTTCTAAAGGTGAAGAATTG** (67 nt)
oIM69[a] reverse	*GTTCTGTATTTTCTTTTACATTCATTTAC***TTATTTATACAATTCATCCATAC[sp] CCAATG** (58 nt)
oIM70[a] forward	**CATTGGGTATGGATGAATTGTATAAATAA***GTAAATGAATGTAA[sp] AAGAAAATACAGAAC* (58 nt)
oIM91 reverse	CTCGATACTGTTCTAGCTTATCTATTTTCTCGG (33 nt)
oIM31 reverse	CAACCAAAATTGGAACAACACC (22 nt)
oIM40 forward	GCTGGTATTACACATGGTATGG (22 nt)
oMB77 forward	CATTGACATGGGGTGTTC (18 nt)
oMB78 reverse	CAATTCATCCATACCCAA (18 nt)
oMB94 forward	GCGCTGCAGGGGTGCAGGA[sp] GGTCAACCTGAGGTTGGTCGT (40 nt)
oMB97 reverse	CCAGGGATCCCGAACATC[sp] TATAATGACCTTATCCGTT (37 nt)
rpsL_3 forward	TGACATGGATACGGAAGTAG (20 nt)
rpsL_4 reverse	ATGGTAAGCTGAGTTATAGC (20 nt)

[a]*Italics* show sequence hybridizing with chromosomal DNA *ftsZ* region
Bold shows sequence hybridizing with *mTurquoise* DNA orf
Underline shows linker sequence

3 Methods

3.1 Generation of a Synthetic Chimeric* ftsZ-mTurquoise *DNA Fragment (See Note 3)

The different steps of the overlapping fusion PCR procedure are shown in Fig. 2.

1. Design three pairs of primers to amplify the 1 kb upstream region of *ftsZ* and the *ftsZ* gene (oIM90-forward and oIM67-

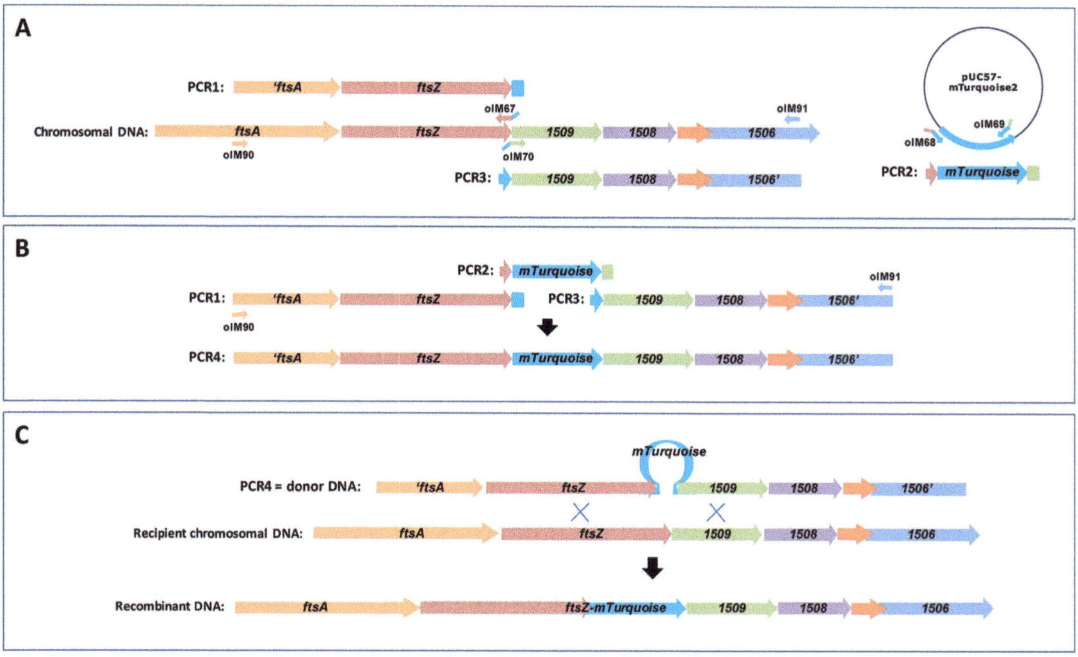

Fig. 2 Illustration of the construction of a strain containing the chimeric translational FtsZ-mTurquoise2 fusion. (**a**) The first step PCR allows amplification of the 2-kb regions flanking the target locus and the fragment carrying the 720-bp heterologous sequence. PCR1 (upstream region) is generated using oIM90 and oIM67; PCR3 (downstream region) is generated using oIM70 and oIM91 and PCR2 (*mTurquoise2 orf*) is generated using oIM68 and oIM69 as indicated. (**b**) The second step PCR was performed using PCR1, PCR2, and PCR3 as templates with outer primers, oIM90 and oIM91 to add the two *ftsZ* regions at the 5′- and 3′-end of the *mTurquoise2 orf*. (**c**) Introduction of the chimeric translational fusion into the *ftsZ* locus by recombination. The PCR4 product is used as the donor DNA for transformation without selection

reverse for PCR1), the *mTurquoise orf* (oIM68-forward and oIM69-reverse for PCR2), and the 2 kb downstream region of *ftsZ* (oIM70-forward and oIM91-reverse for PCR3) (*see* **Notes 4** and **5**).

2. Amplify PCR1 (2077 bp), PCR2 (720 bp), and PCR3 (2036 bp) fragments (*see* **Note 6**) using the high fidelity DNA polymerase, Phusion (ThermoScientific) according to the manufacturer's guidelines.

   Reaction setup (50 μL): Phusion Buffer HF (1×); forward-primer (0.5 μM); reverse-primer (0.5 μM); dNTP (200 μM); chromosomal DNA R304 (2 ng μL^{-1}) or plasmid DNA pUC57-mTurquoise (0.4 ng μL^{-1}); Phusion DNA Polymerase (2 U/50 μL).

   Thermocycling conditions: initial denaturation: 98 °C 30 s—25 cycles: 98 °C 10 s/52 °C 30 s/72 °C 1 min—Final extension: 72 °C 10 min.

3. Examine the resulting PCR amplicons by agarose gel electrophoresis and purify them from the gel using a DNA purification kit (*see* **Note 7**).
4. Amplify the chimeric translational fusion *ftsZ-mTurquoise* (PCR4) using the outer primers, oIM90-forward and oIM91-reverse and equimolar quantities of purified PCR1, PCR2, and PCR3 as template (*see* **Note 8**).

   Reaction setup (50 μL): Phusion Buffer HF (1×); oIM90-forward (0.5 μM); oIM91-reverse (0.5 μM); dNTP (200 μM); equimolar mix of the three PCR products (10 ng μL^{-1} each); Phusion DNA Polymerase (2 U/50 μL).

   Thermocycling conditions: initial denaturation: 98 °C 30 s—25 cycles: 98 °C 10 s/52 °C 30 s/72 °C 5 min—Final extension: 72 °C 10 min.
5. Examine amplicons by agarose gel electrophoresis. Purify the resulting PCR product (4833 bp) corresponding to the chimeric translational fusion *ftsZ-mTurquoise* and the region downstream of *ftsZ* from the gel using a DNA purification kit (*see* **Note 9**).

3.2 Preparation of Precompetent Cells

This step is critical to achieving high transformation efficiency (*see* **Note 10**) [8].

1. Preculture preparation: inoculate acidified C+Y medium (pH adjusted 6.8–7 with 20 mM HCl) with a 1/50 dilution (~6×10^6 cells mL^{-1}) of R1502 stock culture (*see* **Note 11**) and incubate at 37 °C until OD_{550} ~ 0.3 (mid-exponential phase of growth, ~3×10^8 cells mL^{-1}).
2. Dilute preculture 50-fold in acidified C+Y medium and incubate at 37 °C until OD_{550} ~ 0.10 to 0.15 (beginning of exponential growth phase).
3. Harvest cells by centrifugation at 2900 × *g* for 5 min at 4°C.
4. Discard the supernatant and resuspend the pellet in 1/10th volume of C+Y medium complemented by 15% (vol/vol) glycerol.
5. Store as 100 μL samples at −70 °C until required. A 100 μL aliquot is sufficient for ten transformations done in parallel.

3.3 Markerless ftsZ-mTurquoise Recombinant Strain Construction

1. Activation of competence: Thaw a 100 μL aliquot of pre-competent cells on ice. Add 900 μL of C+Y medium (pH 7.8 to 8) containing synthetic CSP (25 to 100 ng mL^{-1}) to the pre-competent cells (*see* **Note 12**). Incubate at 37 °C for 8 min (*see* **Note 13**).
2. DNA internalization: Add purified chimeric *ftsZ-mTurquoise* fragment (saturating concentration >100 ng mL^{-1}) to 100 μL of competence-activated cells and incubate at 30 °C

for 20 min. In parallel, transformation efficiency is measured by transforming the same cell preparation with a selectable donor DNA (*see* **Note 14**).

3. Phenotypic expression: Add 1.4 mL of C+Y medium to 100 μL of transformed cells. Incubate for 4 h at 37 °C (*see* **Note 15**)
4. Make tenfold serial dilutions of the grown cells up to 10^{-6} and plate appropriate dilutions (100 μL of 10^{-5} and 100 μL of 10^{-6}) on petri dishes. Pour 10 mL CAT-agar supplemented with 4% (vol/vol) horse blood on top of the dilutions and mix by gentle agitation to cover the dish. Incubate overnight at 37 °C until colonies become visible.
5. Pick colonies from the agar plate and inoculate one colony per well in a 96-well plate containing 200 μL of C+Y medium in each well. Include an uninoculated C+Y medium negative control. Incubate for 3–4 h at 37 °C (until the medium becomes cloudy). Add glycerol to a final concentration of 15% for storage at −70 °C.

   The number of clones analyzed depends on the efficiency of transformation and on the length of the flanking homologous regions; the yield of recombinants from donor amplicons varies over a 10,000-fold range for homologous arms between 100 and 2000 bp [9] (*see* **Note 16**).
6. Screen clones by PCR for the presence of the heterologous mTurquoise2 *orf* using the pair of primers oIM68-forward and oIM69-reverse. Perform PCR in a 96-well PCR plate using 1 μL from each culture in 20 μL PCR-amplification reaction. Include a negative control (C+Y medium) and a positive control (using a plasmid or a chromosomal DNA template containing the *mTurquoise orf*).

   Reaction setup (20 μL): DreamTaq Green Buffer (1×); oIM68-forward (0.5 μM); oIM69-reverse (0.5 μM); dNTP (200 μM); 1 μL of bacterial culture; DreamTaq DNA Polymerase (2 U/50 μL) (*see* **Note 17**).

   Thermocycling conditions: Initial denaturation: 95 °C 2 min—30 cycles: 95 °C 30 s/55 °C 30 s/72 °C 1 min—Final extension: 72 °C 10 min.

   Analyze the PCR products by agarose gel electrophoresis.
7. Dilute positive recombinant cultures 200-fold in 3 mL acidified C+Y medium and incubate for ~4 to 5 h at 37 °C (OD_{550} ~ 0.3) (*see* **Note 18**).
8. Make tenfold serial dilutions to 10^{-5} and plate dilutions (100 μL of 10^{-5}) on petri dishes. Pour 10 mL CAT-agar supplemented with 4% (vol/vol) horse blood on top of the dilutions and mix by gentle agitation to cover the dish. Incubate overnight at 37 °C.

9. Recover at least two subclones and grow stock cultures in 2.5 mL of THY medium. Incubate for ~ 4 to 5 h at 37 °C (OD_{550} ~ 0.3).
10. Perform a set of PCR screens to validate the construction using the pair of primers oIM90-forward + oIM91-reverse to encompass the chimeric locus; the two pairs of primers oIM90-forward + oIM69-reverse and oIM68-forward + oIM91-reverse to check the border between target gene, *ftsZ* and the *mTurquoise orf* and the upstream or downstream flanking regions of the *ftsZ* gene (*see* **Note 19**). Use the conditions described above (same reaction (DreanTaq polymerase) and same program).
11. Sequence the new region using the amplicon encompassing the complete region (oIM90-forward + oIM91-reverse) and several primers distributed throughout the sequence to verify the integrity of the *ftsZ* and the *mTurquoise* genes, the junctions between these genes, and the downstream region of *ftsZ* fused to the *mTurquoise orf* (i.e., oIM90, oMB94, oIM31, oMB77, oMB78, oIM40, oMB97, and oIM91) (verification of both DNA strands).
12. Check the expression, integrity, and stability of the chimeric translational fusion by western blotting. Other phenotypic analyses could be performed, such as monitoring growth or localization (fluorescence microscopy). Since FtsZ is a marker for cell division, we confirmed the functionality of the chimeric translational FtsZ-mTurquoise fusion by monitoring the doubling time of individual growing cells using time-lapse microscopy (as described in [5]—*see* Fig. 1), which was indistinguishable from wild-type cells.

4 Notes

1. Pneumococcal transformation efficiency is optimal in C+Y medium.

   C+Y medium at pH 7.8–8 allows spontaneous competence development. In contrast, C+Y medium at pH 6.8–7 inhibits competence.
2. The C+Y medium is a complex growth medium derived from Tomasz et al. [10], composed of pre-C medium and of a set of supplements. The pre-C medium and supplements are prepared in advance and stored in the dark for up to several months at RT and 4 °C, respectively. The C+Y medium must be prepared just before use.
   (a) pre-C medium composition: L-cysteine hydrochloride (11.25 mg L^{-1}), CH_3COONa (2 g L^{-1}), casein

hydrolysate (5 g L^{-1}), L-tryptophan (6 mg L^{-1}), K_2HPO_4 (8.5 g L^{-1}). Sterilize by heat (124 °C). Store at RT in the dark, usable up to several months after preparation.

(b) Composition of supplements (prepare each solution separately):

- Sodium pyruvate, 2%: Sterilize by filtration 0.22 μm. Store at 4 °C.
- Bovine serum albumin, 8%: Sterilize by filtration 0.22 μm. Store at 4 °C.
- $MnCl_2{\cdot}4H_2O$, 0.4 mM: Prepare a 0.4 M solution, sterilize by filtration 0.22 μm. Dilute this solution 1000 times and sterilize by filtration 0.22 μm. Store at 4 °C.
- Uridine, 2 mg mL^{-1}/adenosine, 2 mg mL^{-1}: Sterilize by filtration 0.22 μm. Store at 4 °C.
- Sucrose, $C_{12}H_{22}O_{11}$, 50%: Sterilize by heat (110 °C). Store at 4 °C.
- Glucose, $C_6H_{12}O_6$, 20%: Sterilize by heat (110 °C). Store at 4 °C.
- ADAMS I: biotin, $C_{10}H_{16}N_2O_3S$: 0.15 mg L^{-1} (prepare a solution at 0.5 mg mL^{-1} in H_2Omq and add 0.3 mL L^{-1}); nicotinic acid, $C_6H_5NO_2$: 150 mg L^{-1}; pyridoxine hydrochloride, $C_8H_{11}NO_3{\cdot}HCl$: 175 mg L^{-1}; calcium pantothenate, $C_{18}H_{32}N_2O_{10}$: 600 mg L^{-1}; thiamine hydrochloride, $C_{12}H_{17}ClN_4OS{\cdot}HCl$: 160 mg L^{-1}; riboflavin, $C_{17}H_{20}N_4O_6$: 70 mg L^{-1}.

  Dissolve in 1 L of H_2Omq complemented with ~2 mL of NaOH 1 N to adjust the pH to 7.0. Sterilize in boiling water during 15 min. Store (10× 100 mL) at 4 °C in the dark (protect each flask with aluminum foil).
- ADAMS II: iron(II) sulfate, $FeSO_4{\cdot}7H_2O$: 5 g L^{-1}; zinc sulfate, $ZnSO_4{\cdot}7H_2O$: 5 g L^{-1}; copper(II) sulfate, $CuSO_4{\cdot}5H_2O$: 5 g L^{-1}; manganese chloride, $MnCl_2{\cdot}4H_2O$: 2 g L^{-1}. Dissolve in 1 L of H_2Omq complemented of 100 mL of HCl 12 N. Sterilize in boiling water during 15 min. Store (10 × 100 mL) at 4 °C in the dark (protect each flask with aluminum foil).
- ADAMS III: ADAMS I: 130 mL L^{-1}; ADAMS II: 4 mL L^{-1}; L-asparagine·H_2O: 1.6 g L^{-1}; choline chloride, $C_2H_{14}NOCl$: 200 mg L^{-1}; calcium chloride,

$CaCl_2{\cdot}2H_2O$: 0.5 g L^{-1}; magnesium chloride, $MgCl_2{\cdot}6H_2O$: 20 g L^{-1}.

Dissolve in 1 L of H_2Omq. Add ~1 mL of NaOH 6 N to adjust pH to 7.6. Sterilize by filtration 0.22 μm. Store (20 × 50 mL) at 4 °C in the dark (protect each flask with aluminum foil).

- Yeast extract (YE), 10%: Weigh 40 g of yeast extract and add 360 mL of H_2Omq then add 6 mL of HCl 12 N to reduce pH to 3. Carefully, add 16 g of active charcoal, mix gently and incubate for 2 h at 4 °C.

  Filter on a Celite stratum (Celite deposited on Whatman paper on a porcelain filtration unit and wet with H_2Omq) and repeat this step on the same Celite. Add 7 mL of fresh NaOH 10 N (to obtain a pH of ~7.8 to 8) and adjust the volume to 400 mL with H_2Omq. Sterilize by filtration 0.45 μm. Store as 50 mL samples at −20 °C until required. After defrosting, sterilize again by filtration 0.22 μm and store at 4 °C.

  We note that the quality of YE is not always the same depending on suppliers. We therefore advise to always use the same products.

- L-Glutamine, 3%: Sterilize by filtration 0.22 μm. Store at 4 °C. This is optional. It was included historically to complement the growth of *ami* mutants [11].

(c) 100 mL C+Y medium preparation:

- 90 mL of pre-C medium
- 0.1 mL $MnCl_2$ 0.4 mM (250 μg L^{-1} final).
- 0.065 mL sucrose 50% (0.3 g L^{-1} final).
- 0.075 mL L-glutamine 3% (22 mg L^{-1} final).
- 1 mL uridine/adenosine 2 mg/mL (20 mg L^{-1} final).
- 1 mL BSA 8% (0.8 g L^{-1} final).
- 1 mL glucose 20% (2 g L^{-1} final).
- 1.5 mL pyruvic acid 2% (0.3 g L^{-1} final).
- 2.5 mL ADAMS III.
- 2.5 mL yeast extract 10% (25 g L^{-1} final)

  The final pH is to 7.8–8 (ready to use for transformation).

  See Table 2 for suppliers & references and Table 3 for other quantities preparation.

3. Description of *mTurquoise2* and *ftsZ* genes.

   The mTurquoise2 fluorochrome is a variant of mCFP (cyan fluorescent protein), which itself derives from mGFP (green fluorescent protein) [12]. Five amino acid modifications were

Table 2
Alphabetical list of chemicals used to prepare media described in this study

Product	Supplier and reference
Active carbon/charcoal	MERCK—ref.: 102186
Adenosine, $C_{10}H_{13}N_5O_4$	SIGMA—ref.: A-9251
Bacto Casitone	BD—ref.: 225930
Bacto Todd Hewitt	BD—ref.: 249240
Bacto tryptone	BD—ref.: 211705
Biotine $C_{10}H_{16}N_2O_3S$	SIGMA—ref.: B4501
Bovine serum albumin	SIGMA—ref.: A7906
Calcium chloride, $CaCl_2{\cdot}2H_2O$	MERCK—ref.: TA343182
Calcium pantothenate, $C_{18}H_{32}N_2O_{10}$	SIGMA—ref.: P2250
Casein hydrolysate for microbiology	MERCK— 1.022.45.0500
Celite 545	SIGMA—ref.: 419931
Choline chloride, $C_2H_{14}NOCl$	MERCK—ref.: 1131571
Copper(II) sulfate, $CuSO_4{\cdot}5H_2O$	NORMAPUR—ref.: 23174.290
Dextrose, $C_6H_{12}O_6$	BD—ref.: 215530
Glucose, $C_6H_{12}O_6$	MERCK—ref.: 1.08342.1000
Iron(II) sulfate, $FeSO_4{\cdot}7H_2O$	NORMAPUR—ref.: 24244.232
L-Asparagine. $C_4H_8N_2O_3$	SIGMA—ref.: A0884
L-Cysteine, $C_3H_7NO_2S$	SIGMA—ref.: C7352
L-Glutamine, $C_5H_{10}N_2O_3$	MERCK—ref.: K12733889
L-Tryptophan, $C_{11}H_{12}N_2O_2$	SIGMA—ref.: T8659
Magnesium chloride, $MgCl_2{\cdot}6H_2O$	NORMAPUR—ref.: 25108.295
Manganese chloride, $MnCl_2{\cdot}4H_2O$	NORMAPUR—ref.: 2522.233
Manganese dichloride, $MnCl_2$	NORMAPUR—ref.: 25222.233
Nicotinic acid $C_6H_5NO_2$	SIGMA—ref.: N0761
Potassium phosphate dibasic, K_2HPO_4	PROLABO—ref.: 33612.268
Pyridoxine hydrochloride, $C_8H_{11}NO_3{\cdot}HCl$	SIGMA—ref.: P6280
Riboflavin, $C_{17}H_{20}N_4O_6$	SIGMA—ref.: R9504
Saccharose, $C_{12}H_{22}O_{11}$	MERCK—ref.: 1.07651.1000
Sodium acetate, CH_3COONa	NORMAPUR—ref.: 27652.298
Sodium chloride, NaCl	DUCHEFA—ref.: S0520
Sodium pyruvate, $C_3H_3NaO_3$	SIGMA—ref.: P5280

(continued)

Table 2
(continued)

Product	Supplier and reference
Thiamine hydrochloride, $C_{12}H_{17}ClN_4OS{\cdot}HCl$	SIGMA—ref.: T1270
Trizma base, $NH_2C(CH_2OH)_3$	SIGMA—ref.: T6066
Uridine, $C_9H_{12}N_2O_6$	SIGMA—ref.: U3750
Yeast extract (YE)	BD—ref.: 212750
Zinc sulfate, $ZnSO_4{\cdot}7H_2O$	RECTAPUR—ref.: 29247.292

Table 3
Details of quantities for preparation of different volumes of C+Y medium

C+Y medium	10 mL	20 mL	30 mL	40 mL	50 mL	60 mL	200 mL
Pre-C medium	9 mL	18 mL	27 mL	36 mL	45 mL	54 mL	180 mL
$MnCl_2$	10 μL	20 μL	30 μL	40 μL	50 μL	60 μL	200 μL
Glucose 20%	100 μL	200 μL	300 μL	400 μL	500 μL	600 μL	2 mL
ADAMS III	250 μL	500 μL	750 μL	1 mL	1250 μL	1500 μL	5 mL
Glutamine 3%	7.3 μL	14.6 μL	22 μL	29.2 μL	36.5 μL	44 μL	146 μL
Na pyruvate 2%	150 μL	300 μL	450 μL	600 μL	750 μL	900 μL	3 mL
Saccharose 1.5 M	6.3 μL	12.6 μL	19 μL	25.2 μL	31.5 μL	38 μL	126 μL
Uridine adenosine	100 μL	200 μL	300 μL	400 μL	500 μL	600 μL	2 mL
Albumin 8%	100 μL	200 μL	300 μL	400 μL	500 μL	600 μL	2 mL
Yeast extract	250 μL	500 μL	750 μL	1 mL	1250 μL	1500 μL	5 mL

included in the synthesis: T66S; S73A; I147F; H149D; and S176G compared to mCFP. It also contains the A207K substitution that prevents dimerization [13]. The mTurquoise2 fluorochrome exhibits faster maturation and higher photostability than the mCFP, making it a brighter variant. The gene encoding mTurquoise2 was synthesized with codons optimized for *S. pneumoniae* strain R6 (http://gib.genes.nig.ac.jp/) and cloned into pUC57 by Genscript USA to generate plasmid pUC57-*mTurquoise2(Sp)*, the sequence of which is available upon request.

FtsZ is a GTPase that is structurally similar to eukaryotic tubulin and self-assembles into a ring structure beneath the cytoplasmic membrane at the bacterial division site [14]. FtsZ forms a contractile Z-ring at mid-cell which serves as a scaffold for the other cell division proteins to form the divisome. This protein is present in abundant quantities in the cell (between 3000 and 4000 copies per cell [15]).

4. For efficient overlapping PCRs, reverse primer for PCR1 and forward primer for PCR3 should contain 25 to 30 nucleotides annealing with upstream and downstream flanking region, respectively and a tail of 25 to 30 nucleotides annealing with the sequence to integrate (mTurquoise2 *orf* in this case). Higher yields of overlapping PCR4 are obtained when PCR2 is amplified with entirely complementary primers of reverse primer for PCR1 and forward primer for PCR3.

5. The first pair of primers (oIM90-forward + oIM67-reverse) was designed to amplify the first homologous region of about 2 kb containing the *ftsZ* gene without its STOP codon, a 15 bp linker encoding a five LEGSG amino acids residues and the first 28 bp at the 3′ extremity of the *mTurquoise orf* (for PCR1). The purpose of the linker is to allow mobility between the two proteins and to favor their correct folding.

   The second pair of primers (oIM68-forward + oIM69-reverse) was designed to amplify the *mTurquoise2* fluorochrome gene together with the 28 last bp of the *ftsZ* gene without its STOP codon, the linker at its 5′ extremity and 29 bp of the downstream region of the *ftsZ* gene at its 3′ extremity (for PCR2).

   The third pair of primers (oIM70-forward + oIM91-reverse) was designed to amplify the second chromosomal homologous region corresponding to the *ftsZ* downstream chromosomal region together with the 28 last bp of the 3′ end of the *mTurquoise2 orf* (for PCR3).

   Note that the oIM68-forward primer is entirely complementary to the oIM67-reverse primer and the oIM69-reverse primer is entirely complementary to the oIM70-forward primer.

6. PCR1 and PCR3 require genomic DNA as template. The PCR2 requires DNA carrying the synthetic gene encoding the mTurquoise2 fluorochrome: pUC57-*mTurquoise2* (Sp) plasmid.

7. We recommend purifying the PCR fragments from the gel to eliminate potential contaminating PCR products and primers.

   Caution: Minimize the exposure of the DNA fragment to short-wave UV light to prevent excessive nicking of the fragment.

8. The complementary regions of the three amplicons are linked to each other *via* this fourth PCR. The top strand of the first product (PCR1) can anneal to the bottom strand of the second product (PCR2) at one end (on their 3′ extremities) and the top strand of the third product (PCR3) can anneal to the

bottom strand of the second product but at the other end (on their 5′ extremities).

9. Purification following gel electrophoresis is required since many contaminants are amplified with the chimeric fusion.

10. *S. pneumoniae* strains used in the lab were mostly derived from strains R800 [11] and R1501 (*comC0*) [7]. Acidification of the C+Y medium can be bypassed if cells are genetically modified to avoid spontaneous development of competence, such as *comC0* mutants.

11. Stock cultures of our pneumococcal strains were routinely grown at 37 °C in Todd–Hewitt plus Yeast Extract (THY) medium to OD_{550} ~ 0.3 (~3×10^8 cells mL^{-1}); after addition of 15% (vol/vol) glycerol, stocks were kept at −70 °C.

12. Prepare a stock solution of synthetic CSP to 1 mg mL^{-1} by adding 1 mL of 10 mM Sodium Acetate buffer (pH 5.5) to 1 mg of lyophilized CSP (Millegen—France). Prepare 25 or 100 μg mL^{-1} aliquots by dilution in the same buffer (stock 1000×). Store at −20 °C. Depending on the quality of the CSP synthesis, a final concentration of 25 to 100 ng mL^{-1} is required to fully activate cells.

13. Optimal uptake: our results show that maximal uptake occurs 8 min after CSP addition [16].

14. To directly estimate transformation efficiency, use a 2-kb PCR fragment carrying the *rpsL* gene encoding for the 30S ribosomal subunit S12, with the point mutation *str41* (in its middle) that confers resistance to streptomycin [11]. Amplification is achieved using the pair of primers rpsL-3 and rpsL-4 and chromosomal DNA from the R304 strain [6] as template.

    After phenotypic expression, select transformants by plating appropriate dilutions (100 μL of 10^{-4} to 100 μL of 10^{-6}) on petri dishes. Pour 10 mL CAT-agar supplemented with 4% (vol/vol) horse blood containing streptomycin on top of the dilutions and mix by gentle agitation to cover the dish. To measure the total number of cells, plate appropriate dilutions (100 μL of 10^{-5} and 100 μL of 10^{-6}) on petri dishes. Pour 10 mL CAT-agar supplemented with 4% (vol/vol) horse blood. Incubate overnight at 37 °C.

    With a 2-kb *str41* PCR fragment (using saturating concentrations: 100 to 200 ng mL^{-1}), expected transformation efficiency is between 80% to 100%.

    The next screening step of ftsZ-mTurquoise2 transformants should not be performed if the transformation efficiency is lower.

15. These dilution and growth steps allow segregation of pure transformants.

16. The number of clones analyzed depends on the size of the flanking homologous regions and to a lesser extent on the size of the heterologous fragment integrated. Indeed, a donor DNA fragment containing ~1-kb homologous sequences flanking a 720 bp heterologous region required the screening of 100 clones to recover 1 to 5% positive transformants.

    In contrast, 20 clones were sufficient to recover positive transformants (10% to 20%) when a donor fragment containing ~2-kb homologous flanking regions was used.

    However, increasing the size of the homologous amplified regions (>2-kb) increases the risk of integrating point mutations in amplicons. We therefore recommend to not exceeding 2-kb of homology on both sides of the integrated DNA.

    Alternative procedure for strains that transform poorly: Screen at least 200 clones: inoculate 20 tubes containing 2 mL of acidified C+Y medium with 10 independent colonies each and incubate for 4 h at 37 °C. Use 1 μL of this culture in 20 μL PCR reactions mixtures. Then proceed with the steps described for the isolation and verification of positive transformants.
17. Prepare a mix with all components except the culture, distribute in each well, and then add the culture. (For convenience, use a multichannel pipette with either 8 or 12 channels.)
18. To isolate recombinants from the positive clones obtained, carry out a new round of segregation. Indeed, the chaining growth habit of streptococci is likely to ensure that colonies recovered soon after transformation could be mixed with wild-type cells and cells harboring the chimeric construct [17].
19. In the case of pure transformant clones, only one product is expected with the pair of primers oIM90-forward + oIM91-reverse. However, if the clone is mixed (recombinants and parental cells), two products are amplified.

    With the pairs of primers oIM90-forward + oIM69-reverse and oIM68-forward + oIM91-reverse, there is no amplification if the integration is not in the *ftsZ* chromosomal locus.

Acknowledgments

We warmly thank Jean-Pierre Claverys and Bernard Martin for their prominent contribution to development of pneumococcal genetics. We thank Dave Lane and Calum Johnston for critical reading of the manuscript. We also thank all past members of the Claverys lab, past and present members of the Polard lab who participated in development of the method. This work was funded by the Centre

National de la Recherche Scientifique, Université Paul Sabatier and Agence Nationale de la Recherche (Grant ANR-13-BSV8-0022 and ANR-17-CE13-0031).

References

1. Sung CK, Li H, Claverys JP, Morrison DA (2001) An rpsL cassette, janus, for gene replacement through negative selection in Streptococcus pneumoniae. Appl Environ Microbiol 67:5190–5196. https://doi.org/10.1128/AEM.67.11.5190-5196.2001
2. Weng L, Biswas I, Morrison DA (2009) A self-deleting Cre-lox-ermAM cassette, Cheshire, for marker-less gene deletion in Streptococcus pneumoniae. J Microbiol Methods 79:353–357. https://doi.org/10.1016/j.mimet.2009.10.007
3. Iannelli F, Pozzi G (2004) Method for introducing specific and unmarked mutations into the chromosome of Streptococcus pneumoniae. Mol Biotechnol 26:81–86. https://doi.org/10.1385/MB:26:1:81
4. Junges R, Khan R, Tovpeko Y et al (2017) Markerless genome editing in competent streptococci. Methods Mol Biol 1537:233–247. https://doi.org/10.1007/978-1-4939-6685-1_14
5. Bergé MJ, Mercy C, Mortier-Barrière I et al (2017) A programmed cell division delay preserves genome integrity during natural genetic transformation in Streptococcus pneumoniae. Nat Commun 8:1621. https://doi.org/10.1038/s41467-017-01716-9
6. Mortier-Barrière I, de Saizieu A, Claverys JP, Martin B (1998) Competence-specific induction of recA is required for full recombination proficiency during transformation in Streptococcus pneumoniae. Mol Microbiol 27:159–170
7. Dagkessamanskaia A, Moscoso M, Hénard V et al (2004) Interconnection of competence, stress and CiaR regulons in Streptococcus pneumoniae: competence triggers stationary phase autolysis of ciaR mutant cells. Mol Microbiol 51:1071–1086
8. Prudhomme M, Attaiech L, Sanchez G et al (2006) Antibiotic stress induces genetic transformability in the human pathogen Streptococcus pneumoniae. Science 313:89–92. https://doi.org/10.1126/science.1127912
9. Lau PCY, Sung CK, Lee JH et al (2002) PCR ligation mutagenesis in transformable streptococci: application and efficiency. J Microbiol Methods 49:193–205
10. Tomasz A (1967) Choline in the cell wall of a bacterium: novel type of polymer-linked choline in pneumococcus. Science 157:694–697
11. Lefevre JC, Claverys JP, Sicard AM (1979) Donor deoxyribonucleic acid length and marker effect in pneumococcal transformation. J Bacteriol 138:80–86
12. Mérola F, Fredj A, Betolngar D-B et al (2014) Newly engineered cyan fluorescent proteins with enhanced performances for live cell FRET imaging. Biotechnol J 9:180–191. https://doi.org/10.1002/biot.201300198
13. Zacharias DA, Violin JD, Newton AC, Tsien RY (2002) Partitioning of lipid-modified monomeric GFPs into membrane microdomains of live cells. Science 296:913–916. https://doi.org/10.1126/science.1068539
14. Bi EF, Lutkenhaus J (1991) FtsZ ring structure associated with division in *Escherichia coli*. Nature 354:161–164. https://doi.org/10.1038/354161a0
15. Jacq M, Adam V, Bourgeois D et al (2015) Remodeling of the Z-ring nanostructure during the Streptococcus pneumoniae cell cycle revealed by Photoactivated localization microscopy. MBio 6:e01108-15. https://doi.org/10.1128/mBio.01108-15
16. Bergé MJ, Kamgoué A, Martin B et al (2013) Midcell recruitment of the DNA uptake and virulence nuclease, EndA, for pneumococcal transformation. PLoS Pathog 9:e1003596. https://doi.org/10.1371/journal.ppat.1003596
17. Morrison DA, Khan R, Junges R et al (2015) Genome editing by natural genetic transformation in Streptococcus mutans. J Microbiol Methods 119:134–141. https://doi.org/10.1016/j.mimet.2015.09.023

Chapter 7

Gene Expression Analysis in the Pneumococcus

Rory A. Eutsey, Carol A. Woolford, Surya D. Aggarwal, Rolando A. Cuevas, and N. Luisa Hiller

Abstract

Bacterial cells modify their gene expression profiles throughout different stages of growth and in response to environmental cues. Analyses of gene expression across conditions reveal both conserved and condition-specific gene responses of bacteria to adapt to these dynamic conditions. In this chapter, we present a guide to pneumococcal RNA extraction for use in the NanoString nCounter platform. The nCounter is a highly effective method to measure gene expression of bacteria not only in a planktonic mode of growth but also in the presence of host cells where the RNA of interest represents only a small portion of the total material.

Key words RNA isolation, Gene expression, Transcriptome, NanoString

1 Introduction

Gene expression profiling has long been performed to understand the biology and pathogenesis of the human pathogen *Streptococcus pneumoniae*. Numerous studies have applied qRT-PCR to dissect the expression of small sets of genes [1–5]. Further, microarrays covering the whole genome of model strains or the majority of the genes in the pneumococcal pangenome have been widely applied for a comprehensive view of gene expression [6–12]. These transcriptomic studies have greatly enhanced our understanding of gene regulation in the pneumococcus. The current challenge is to measure gene expression of pneumococci grown in vivo. RNAseq and NanoString are technologies that address this gap [11–15]. Here, we present protocols for RNA extraction and processing using the NanoString nCounter platform (Fig. 1) [16]. Our protocols address planktonic cells, in vitro biofilms grown on epithelial cells, middle-ear effusion from the chinchilla model of otitis media, and lungs from the murine model of pneumonia.

Federico Iovino (ed.), *Streptococcus pneumoniae: Methods and Protocols*, Methods in Molecular Biology, vol. 1968, https://doi.org/10.1007/978-1-4939-9199-0_7,

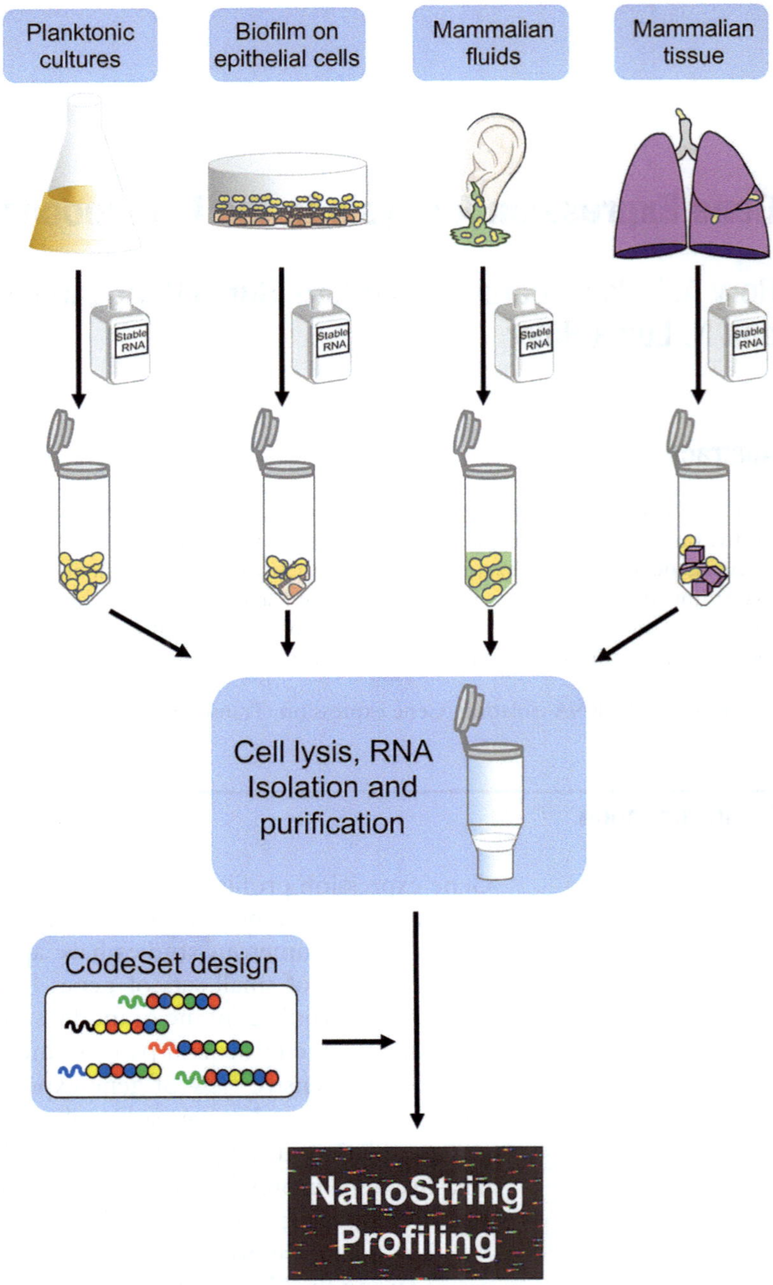

Fig. 1 Schematic of RNA Analysis using the NanoString. This chapter focuses on sample preparation, pneumococcal cell lysis, RNA extraction and purification, and NanoString profiling

2 Materials

2.1 Sample Preservation

1. Liquid Nitrogen.
2. RNAprotect Cell Reagent (Qiagen) or RNAlater Stabilization Solution (Thermo).
3. In-house RNA stabilization solution: 5.3 M ammonium sulfate, 20 mM EDTA, 25 mM sodium citrate in distilled water.

2.2 Lysis of Pneumococcal Cells

1. Lysozyme: dissolved in distilled water to 100 mg/ml.
2. Mutanolysin: dissolved in distilled water to 200 μg/ml.
3. Proteinase K: dissolved in distilled water to 20 mg/ml.
4. Tris EDTA buffer (TE). 100× concentrate: 1 M Tris–HCl pH 8, 0.1 M EDTA-Na_2.
5. Lysis Solution. For 200 μl add 128 μl TE buffer, 27 μl lysozyme, 27 μl mutanolysin, and 18 μl proteinase K. For 800 μl add 512 μl TE buffer, 108 μl lysozyme, 108 μl mutanolysin, and 72 μl proteinase K.
6. Zirconia/silica beads 0.5 mm in diameter.
7. GentleMACS dissociator.
8. GentleMACS M tubes.
9. Acid-phenol–chloroform 5:1 at pH 4.5.
10. Nuclease-free water.

2.3 RNA Extraction and Purification

1. Column-based RNA extraction kit.
   (a) Quick-RNA MiniPrep kit (Zymo Research).
   (b) RNeasy Mini kit (Qiagen).
   (c) PureLink RNA Mini kit (Invitrogen).
2. DNase (Turbo DNase (Invitrogen)).

2.4 RNA Quantification

1. Spectrophotometer (NanoDrop).

3 Methods

3.1 Sample Preservation

3.1.1 Planktonic Cultures

1. Grow pneumococcal cells in a liquid culture in a conical tube (*see* **Note 1** for details on growth conditions).

   We routinely use 10^8–10^9 cells, which provide an estimated 10–100 μg of RNA. The stage of growth and volume required to collect this number of cells will depend on experimental goals.
2. To the culture, add either 2 volumes of RNAprotect Bacteria reagent or 1 volume of in-house RNA stabilization solution.

3. Centrifuge samples at 4000 × *g* for 10 min to pellet cells.
4. Discard the supernatant.
5. Freeze cell pellet at −80 °C in the conical tubes.

3.1.2 In Vitro Biofilms on Epithelial Cells

1. Grow biofilms in cell culture flasks (*see* Subheading 4 on growth conditions).
2. Remove media from cell culture flask, using care to avoid dispersion of the biofilm.
3. Add RNAlater bacteria reagent or in-house RNA stabilization solution until the cells on the bottom of the flask are completely immersed.
4. Scrape the bottom of the flask with a cell sterile cell scraper to release the bacterial cells, use a pipette to remove all material from the flask and collect the biofilm material into a conical tube.
5. Centrifuge at 4000 × *g* for 10 min to pellet the cells.
6. Discard the supernatant.
7. Freeze cells pellet at −80 °C in the conical tube.

3.1.3 Infected Mammalian Tissue (Soft Tissue)[1]

1. Collect the tissue of interest from the animal, place in a microfuge tube (without any liquid).
2. *Immediately* flash-freeze the sample by placing the microfuge tube in liquid nitrogen.
3. Store sample at −80 °C.

3.1.4 Infected Mammalian Fluids (Effusions)[1]

1. Collect effusion fluids from chinchilla middle ears and place in a microfuge tube (*see* **Note 2** for details).
2. *Immediately* flash-freeze the sample by placing the microfuge tube in liquid nitrogen.
3. Store sample at −80 °C.

3.2 Sample Lysis[2]

3.2.1 Planktonic Cultures and In Vitro Biofilms on Epithelial Culture

1. Prepare the lysis solution. Each sample will require 200 μl of lysis solution.
2. Remove sample from freezer and thaw at RT.
3. Add 200 μl lysis solution to the cell pellet.

---

[1] In our initial RNA extractions from murine tissue, we employed RNAlater to preserve RNA (Life Technologies) and observed very low yields. Our yields improved with flash-freezing the tissue immediately after removal from the animal.

[2] We lyse cells at room temperature, and have found that we achieved high quality RNA (as measured by an Agilent Bioanalyzer). However, many laboratories maintain material on ice while extracting RNA. We elected room temperature, to ensure full activity of the cell wall lytic enzymes.

4. Resuspend the pellet and incubate at room temperature for 20 min, while vortexing every 5 min.
5. Proceed to "RNA Extraction and Purification."

3.2.2 Infected Mammalian Tissue Samples (This Protocol Has Been Used for Murine Lungs)

1. Prepare the following: gentleMACS M tube, tissue lysis solution, and 15 ml conical tube.
2. Remove sample from freezer and thaw at room temperature.
3. Move the tissue sample, weighing no more than 150 mg, to a gentleMACS M tube. Add 800 μl lysis solution.
4. To homogenize the tissue, place the tube in the gentleMACS dissociator and run the preset RNA protocol RNA_02.01 (*see* **Note 3** for an alternative).
5. Incubate the material in the M tube at room temperature for 20 min to allow lysis of the bacterial cell wall. At this point, the solution will be cloudy with a reddish color.
6. Remove all liquid (~800 μl) from the M tube and place into a 15 ml conical tube.
7. Proceed to "RNA Extraction and Purification."

3.2.3 Infected Mammalian Fluids (This Protocol Has Been Used for Chinchilla Middle-Ear Effusions)

1. Prepare the following: 1.5 ml screw-cap microcentrifuge tube with 0.5 mm zirconia/silica beads, cell lysis solution, and 1.5 ml microcentrifuge tube.
2. Remove sample from freezer and thaw at room temperature.
3. Mix 200 μl of effusion with 14 μl of TE, 14 μl lysozyme, 14 μl of mutanolysin, and 9 μl proteinase K in a 1.5 ml screw-cap microcentrifuge tube with an estimated 100 μl of 0.5 mm zirconia/silica beads.
4. Incubate at room temperature for 10 min.
5. Bead-beat twice, for 30 s each.
6. Incubate at room temperature for 10 min.
7. Remove the liquid (leaving beads behind, as they settle to the bottom) and transfer to a 1.5 ml microcentrifuge tube.
8. Proceed to 'RNA Extraction and Purification'.

3.3 RNA Extraction and Purification

This step is the same for all samples described above.

1. Perform RNA extraction and purification using a column-based RNA mini prep kit following the specific manufacturer's instructions. We use the Quick-RNA MiniKit from Zymo (however other kits should also work). Scale the prep for the amount of starting liquid material. Specifically: 200 μl for planktonic cultures, 200 μl for biofilms, 800 μl for solid tissue samples, and 200 μl for body fluids.

2. For NanoString analysis, samples do not need to be DNA-free. NanoString probes only hybridize to single-stranded targets, and the sample hybridization and processing steps do not result in DNA denaturation. Thus, there is no need for DNA removal beyond the one provided by the kit.
3. Quantify the RNA. To this end, use a spectrophotometer, such as a NanoDrop. The purity of the sample can be estimated by calculating the 260/280 absorbance ratio, where pure RNA will have a ratio around 2.0.

3.4 CodeSet Design

Design the CodeSet in conjunction with the NanoString team. CodeSet reagents and cartridges are designed for 12 samples to be run at one time. Considerations are listed below.

1. First select the RNA transcripts of interest for your experiment. Currently CodeSets can be designed to detect from 20 to 800 transcripts. Each probe is 100 bp long.
2. Include multiple normalization controls in the CodeSet. We recommend at least two housekeeping genes that have little to no variability in expression across all treatment conditions. Optimally, genes used for normalization controls should have levels of abundance in the range of the experimental genes. Normalization is performed on the geometric mean of these controls. We consistently use *gyrB* (DNA gyrase, B subunit, SPD_0709) and *metG* (methionyl-tRNA synthetase, SPD_0689). For experiments within related conditions we also use *gapdh* (glyceraldehyde-3-phosphate dehydrogenase, SPD_1004); however, we do not recommend this control to compare across diverse modes of growth (such as planktonic versus biofilms or in vitro versus in vivo). Do not use 16S rRNA, as the high abundance of this gene will cover a high proportion of the field of view, resulting in suboptimal data (Subheading 3.5).
3. We consistently capture a range of probe signals of five orders of magnitude. That is, RNA reads range from single digits to a few hundred thousand counts for a single molecule. However, if interested in very low-abundance transcripts, consider designing a CodeSet with only low-abundance transcripts.
4. Include positive controls using genes induced in the condition of interest. For in vivo conditions, we use *ply* (pneumolysin, SPD_1726) and *vp1* (virulence peptide 1, SPD_0145) [17].
5. Consider specificity. For studies in the presence of host cells, avoid probes that can cross-react to host molecules.
6. Consider strain variation. If multiple pneumococcal strains will be tested, design probes to conserved regions of the transcript, so that they capture allelic variants. In general, 95% identity to the target sequence is sufficient to ensure binding. This step

can be performed in collaboration with the NanoString team and/or using BLASTn. With BLASTn, generate a database with all the alleles of interest and select probes that recognize each and every sequence with at least 95% identity over the length of the entire probe.

3.5 Estimation of RNA Amount

Establish the amount of RNA for each sample. Note that during data acquisition, the probe–transcript complexes are immobilized on the nCounter cartridge, imaged, and enumerated. For successful quantification, the binding density on the cartridge must be within an acceptable range (varies with nCounter instrument; 0.05–2.25 for Gen1 nCounter and 0.1–1.8 for the nCounter SPRINT, per manufacturer's instructions). That is, there must be sufficient RNA to allow statistically relevant counts of the transcripts of interest but not so much material that the field of view (FOV) is saturated and single molecules cannot be discerned. The transcripts of interest may correspond to a high percentage of the total RNA (in a pure planktonic culture), or a very small percentage when bacteria are mixed with mammalian tissue. Thus, the optimal starting RNA concentration is highly dependent on the percentage of the transcript of interest relative to total RNA. It will also depend on the number of probes in the CodeSet and abundance of the targets within the species of interest. In this session, we provide empirical information collected over our experiments. In all cases, the final volume of RNA is set at a maximum of 5 μl.

1. For pure planktonic cultures, where all the RNA is from pneumococcus, dilute the samples to a concentration of approximately 10–15 ng/μl, for an estimated total of 50–75 ng of RNA per experiment. This has been successful for CodeSets ranging from 50 to 200 targets. In contrast, experiments performed with ten times this concentration were not interpretable due to higher-than-optimal binding density and image saturation.
2. For pneumococcal biofilms grown on mammalian epithelial cells, dilute the samples to a concentration of approximately 10–30 ng/μl, for an estimated total of 50–150 ng of total RNA per experiment (*see* Subheading 4 for conditions).
3. For middle-ear effusions, where there is a mix of bacterial and host, do not dilute the RNA. We use RNA at 80–200 ng/μl, for an estimated total of 400–1000 ng of RNA per experiment.
4. For murine lungs, do not dilute the RNA. We estimate that bacterial RNA is <0.1% of total RNA. Thus, we do not dilute the RNA and sometimes concentrated the RNA three- to fourfold. In this case, the optimized concentration will depend on the infection rate of the tissue. As a rule of thumb, we homogenize one lung, and when possible use samples with at least 10^5 CFU/mg of tissue. However, we have found that we

can reach a binding density within the desired range with as little as 3×10^4 CFU/mg of tissue, if we concentrate the material 3–4× by lyophilization. In murine lungs, our nucleic acid concentration ranges from 1000 to 3000 ng/μl before concentration to 15,000 ng/μl after concentration. In a few cases, using very high concentrations has saturated the FOV. Thus, if the CFUs are above 10^5 CFU/mg of tissue we recommend using the RNA from purification, without any further manipulation.

3.6 NanoString Profiling

This is the hybridization protocol for the nCounter XT CodeSet gene expression assays.

1. Remove a tube of reporter CodeSet and Capture ProbeSet reagents from −80 °C freezer and thaw at room temperature. Flick several times and briefly spin down reagents.
2. Create a master mix by adding 70 μl hybridization buffer to the Reporter CodeSet tube. Invert repeatedly and spin down gently.
3. Add 8 μl master mix to each tube in a 0.2 ml thin-wall strip of 12 tubes.
4. Add 5 μl RNA sample or RNA + water to bring up to 5 μl volume.
5. Add 2 μl Capture ProbeSet to each tube, flick briefly, and spin down gently.
6. Immediately place tubes in preheated 65 °C thermocycler and incubate reactions for at least 16 h.

When used in an nCounter SPRINT Profiler, the samples are loaded into a cartridge per manufacturer's instructions and placed in the instrument for sample purification and data collection. Consumable reagents required include cartridges and the nCounter SPRINT Profiler Reagent Pack. Other instrumentation is also available from NanoString for gene expression analysis.

nSolver Analysis Software is available for data analysis following manufacturer's instructions. Software automatically checks data quality and flags samples that are out of the normal range. One can perform technical adjustments such as normalization and determine ratios and differential expression using built-in functions or export data to software of choice.

4 Notes

1. Pneumococcal growth
   (a) Planktonic cultures. For growth in liquid culture, grow colonies from a frozen stock overnight on TSA plates. The

next morning, inoculate colonies into media of choice and incubate at 37 °C and 5% CO_2 without shaking.

(b) Biofilms on epithelial cells. (We employ human type II lung epithelial cell line A549.) Culture cells in DMEM 1× with 4.5 g/l glucose, 8 mM L-glutamine, and 1 mM sodium pyruvate and supplemented with 10% fetal bovine serum containing 20 units/ml of penicillin and 20 μg/ml of streptomycin. Maintain the cell culture on sterile, tissue-culture treated plastic at 37 °C with humidified 5% carbon dioxide atmosphere. Seed epithelial cells at a confluent density of 1×10^6 cells·cm^{-2}. (Confluence is confirmed next day by light microscopy.) Wash the cells with PBS to remove any trace of antibiotic prior to bacterial inoculation. Grow starter cultures of the selected pneumococcal strain to an OD600 of 0.025, then inoculate 100 μl of bacterial cells into the tissue culture plates (estimated 3×10^6 bacteria in total). Incubate plates aerobically in humidified conditions at 37 °C and 5% carbon dioxide for selected time. (We use 16 h.) Before collection, carefully aspirate the supernatants to remove debris, and wash the biofilms with PBS to remove non-adherent and weakly adherent bacteria.

2. Collection of middle-ear effusion from the chinchilla middle ear

   Once the animal has been euthanized, remove the bulla from the chinchilla [18]. Using small surgical scissors, make a minor incision (5 mm diameter) at the top of the bulla. Check for presence of effusion by moving the bulla to sense and view liquid. If there is liquid present, insert a 0.5 ml sterile disposable plastic Pasteur pipette and collect all the effusion (the volume ranges from 50 to 400 μl in a strain and host-dependent manner). If liquid is absent or estimated to be below 50 μl, add 400 μl of PBS, pipet up and down to wash bulla, and collect all liquid.

3. Alternative for tissue homogenizing

   You can homogenize the tissue sample using a bead-beating apparatus. Add the tissue to a 1.5 ml screw-cap tube filled with 100 μl of 0.5 mm zirconia/silica beads.

Acknowledgments

We would like to thank Dr. Aaron Mitchell and Dr. Wenjie Xu for introducing, training, and guiding us in the use of the NanoString technology. We would like to thank Anagha Kadam for performing the first sets of NanoString experiments in our laboratory. We would like to thank Elnaz Ebrahimi for her assistance with growing biofilms on epithelial cells.

References

1. Ogunniyi AD, Giammarinaro P, Paton JC (2002) The genes encoding virulence-associated proteins and the capsule of Streptococcus pneumoniae are upregulated and differentially expressed in vivo. Microbiology 148 (7):2045–2053
2. Ogunniyi AD, Mahdi LK, Trappetti C, Verhoeven N, Mermans D, Van der Hoek MB et al (2012) Identification of genes that contribute to the pathogenesis of invasive pneumococcal disease by in vivo transcriptomic analysis. Infect Immun 80(9):3268–3278
3. Mahdi LK, Deihimi T, Zamansani F, Fruzangohar M, Adelson DL, Paton JC et al (2014) A functional genomics catalogue of activated transcription factors during pathogenesis of pneumococcal disease. BMC Genomics 15(1):769
4. Mahdi LK, Ogunniyi AD, LeMessurier KS, Paton JC (2008) Pneumococcal virulence gene expression and host cytokine profiles during pathogenesis of invasive disease. Infect Immun 76(2):646–657
5. LeMessurier KS, Ogunniyi AD, Paton JC (2006) Differential expression of key pneumococcal virulence genes in vivo. Microbiol Read Engl 152(Pt 2):305–311
6. Tettelin H, Nelson KE, Paulsen IT, Eisen JA, Read TD, Peterson S et al (2001) Complete genome sequence of a virulent isolate of Streptococcus pneumoniae. Science 293 (5529):498–506
7. Orihuela CJ, Radin JN, Sublett JE, Gao G, Kaushal D, Tuomanen EI (2004) Microarray analysis of pneumococcal gene expression during invasive disease. Infect Immun 72 (10):5582–5596
8. Sebert ME, Patel KP, Plotnick M, Weiser JN (2005) Pneumococcal HtrA protease mediates inhibition of competence by the CiaRH two-component signaling system. J Bacteriol 187(12):3969–3979
9. Petersen TN, Brunak S, von Heijne G, Nielsen H (2011) SignalP 4.0: discriminating signal peptides from transmembrane regions. Nat Methods 8(10):785–786
10. Dagkessamanskaia A, Moscoso M, Hénard V, Guiral S, Overweg K, Reuter M et al (2004) Interconnection of competence, stress and CiaR regulons in Streptococcus pneumoniae: competence triggers stationary phase autolysis of ciaR mutant cells. Mol Microbiol 51 (4):1071–1086
11. Kimaro Mlacha SZ, Romero-Steiner S, Hotopp JCD, Kumar N, Ishmael N, Riley DR et al (2013) Phenotypic, genomic, and transcriptional characterization of Streptococcus pneumoniae interacting with human pharyngeal cells. BMC Genomics 14:383
12. Kadam A, Eutsey RA, Rosch J, Miao X, Longwell M, Xu W et al (2017) Promiscuous signaling by a regulatory system unique to the pandemic PMEN1 pneumococcal lineage. PLoS Pathog 13(5):e1006339
13. Cheng S, Clancy CJ, Xu W, Schneider F, Hao B, Mitchell AP et al (2013) Profiling of Candida albicans gene expression during intra-abdominal candidiasis identifies biologic processes involved in pathogenesis. J Infect Dis 208(9):1529–1537
14. Xu W, Solis NV, Ehrlich RL, Woolford CA, Filler SG, Mitchell AP (2015) Activation and alliance of regulatory pathways in C. albicans during mammalian infection. PLoS Biol 13(2): e1002076
15. Xu W, Solis NV, Filler SG, Mitchell AP (2016) Pathogen gene expression profiling during infection using a Nanostring nCounter platform. Methods Mol Biol 1361:57–65
16. Geiss GK, Bumgarner RE, Birditt B, Dahl T, Dowidar N, Dunaway DL et al (2008) Direct multiplexed measurement of gene expression with color-coded probe pairs. Nat Biotechnol 26(3):317–325
17. Cuevas RA, Eutsey R, Kadam A, West-Roberts JA, Woolford CA, Mitchell AP et al (2017) A novel streptococcal cell-cell communication peptide promotes pneumococcal virulence and biofilm formation. Mol Microbiol 105 (4):554–571
18. Giebink GS (1999) Otitis media: the chinchilla model. Microb Drug Resist 5(1):57–72

Chapter 8

Transcriptional Knockdown in Pneumococci Using CRISPR Interference

Morten Kjos

Abstract

Sequence-specific knockdown of gene expression using CRISPR interference (CRISPRi) has recently been developed for *Streptococcus pneumoniae*. By coexpression of a catalytically inactive Cas9-protein (dCas9) and a single guide RNA (sgRNA), CRISPRi can be used to knock down transcription of any gene of interest. Gene specificity is mediated by a 20 bp sequence on the sgRNA, and new genes can be targeted by replacing this 20 bp sequence. Here, a protocol is provided for design of sgRNAs and construction of CRIPSRi strains in *S. pneumoniae*, based on the vectors published by Liu et al. (Mol Syst Biol 13:931, 2017).

Key words CRISPRi, dCas9, Knockdown, sgRNA, Inverse PCR

1 Introduction

Functional studies of essential genes in bacteria rely on construction of depletion or knockdown mutants, since inactivation of such genes is lethal. Knockdown or depletion strains can be constructed by conventional approaches, where an inducible copy of the gene is introduced in an ectopic locus in the chromosome (or on a plasmid), followed by deletion of the native gene. Expression of the essential gene can then be titrated by different inducer concentrations. Another possibility to knock down expression of genes and operons is to utilize the CRISPR/Cas9-based technology known as CRISPR interference (CRISPRi) [1]. With CRISPRi, a catalytically dead Cas9 protein (dCas9) is used to selectively knock down the expression of a gene of interest. Unlike the wild-type Cas9 nuclease, dCas9 does not cleave DNA, but the DNA-binding capability is still intact. A single guide RNA (sgRNA) [2], containing a gene-specific base-pairing region and a structured region for interaction with dCas9, is designed to target the gene of interest. Upon coexpression, the dCas9-sgRNA complex binds DNA close to the 5′ end of the gene and serves as transcriptional roadblock for RNA

Federico Iovino (ed.), *Streptococcus pneumoniae: Methods and Protocols*, Methods in Molecular Biology, vol. 1968, https://doi.org/10.1007/978-1-4939-9199-0_8, © Springer Science+Business Media, LLC, part of Springer Nature 2019

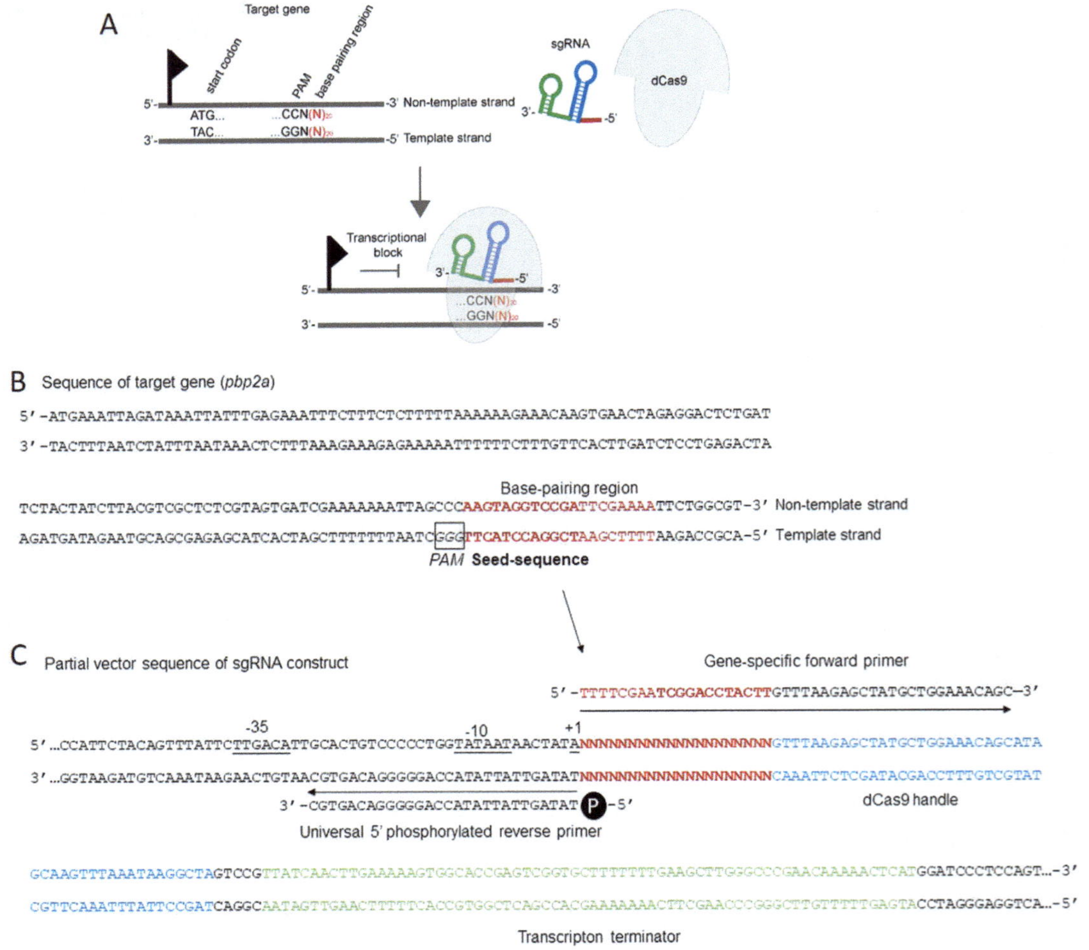

Fig. 1 Overview of the CRISPRi system. (**a**) Schematic overview of CRISPRi. The start codon, PAM-sequence, and base-pairing region of the target genes are shown as well as the sgRNA and dCas9 protein. The promoter is shown as a flag. When sgRNA binds to the nontemplate strand, the DNA-sgRNA-dCas9 complex forms a transcriptional roadblock, causing knockdown of expression of the target gene. (**b** and **c**). Inverse PCR primer design to construct novel sgRNAs, using the pneumococcal gene *pbp2b* as an example. (**b**) The beginning of the *pbp2b*-encoding sequence including start codon ATG. The first PAM site is indicated (box), as well as the base-pairing region (red). The 12 bp seed sequence of the base-pairing region is shown in bold. (**c**) Construction of the sgRNA vector. The base-pairing region is introduced as an overhang on the forward primer, which anneals in the dCas9 handle region. The reverse primer is universal and phosphorylated in the 5′ end to allow ligation of the linearized vector

polymerase, thereby downregulating transcription (Fig. 1). The level of knockdown with CRISPRi can also be titrated by expressing one of the components (dCas9 or sgRNA) from an inducible promoter. A major advantage of CRISPRi over conventional construction of knockdown strains is that new genes can be targeted by a single cloning step; only the 20 nt base-pairing region of the sgRNA constructs needs to be changed to knock down a gene of interest. This allows for construction of large libraries of sgRNA strains [3–5]. On the other hand, a disadvantage with the system is the polar effects when targeting genes within an operon. Since the mechanism involves blocking transcription, all genes downstream of a target gene in an operon will be affected [3].

Streptococcus pneumoniae does not contain an endogenous CRISPR/Cas system [6, 7], and CRISPR/Cas9 can therefore be harnessed for different purposes in this bacterium. Liu et al. [3] recently developed an inducible CRISPRi for *S. pneumoniae*; vectors for chromosomal integration of sgRNA and *dcas9* constructs by double crossover were made. The CRISPRi system was shown to be specific and titratable [3]. In the same work, a library of CRISPRi strains targeting all essential genes in *S. pneumoniae* strain D39 was constructed. The collection comprises approximately 350 strains, which were all phenotypically characterized and eventually used for identifying the function of uncharacterized genes involved in cell wall synthesis and competence development [3]. Also worth noting, CRISPR/Cas9 has also been harnessed for other purposes in *S. pneumoniae*, including introduction of double strand breaks in DNA in strain D39 [8], and to mutagenize genes in *S. pneumoniae* R6 [7].

This chapter explains how an sgRNA should be designed to effectively and specifically target a gene of interest and how the vectors designed by Liu et al. [3] can be used to construct strains for CRISPRi knockdown.

2 Materials

2.1 Related to Design and Construction of New sgRNA Plasmids

1. Genome sequence of your pneumococcal strain.
2. sgRNA template plasmid and sequence: pPEPX-P3-sgRNAluc (Addgene #85590).
3. Universal, 5′ phosphorylated reverse primer (5′-TATAGTTA TTATACCAGGGGGACAGTGC-3′) (*see* **Note 1**).
4. Designed reverse sgRNA primer containing the 20 bp base-pairing sequence.
5. Reagents for high fidelity PCR (Phusion polymerase, dNTPs).
6. Equipment for agarose gel electrophoresis.
7. PCR purification kit.
8. DpnI enzyme and buffer.
9. T4 ligase.
10. *Escherichia coli* cloning host (e.g., DH5α).
11. LB broth (10 g/L NaCl, 10 g/L tryptone, 5 g/L yeast extract).

12. LA agar plates (10 g/L NaCl, 10 g/L tryptone, 5 g/L yeast extract, 1.5% agar) with 100 μg/mL spectinomycin.
13. Plasmid purification kit.
14. Sequencing primer (Ppepx_Seq_R; 5′-CGAGGGATTTGGTG ATTCTTCTT-3′).

2.2 Related to the Construction of CRISPRi Strains

1. Competent pneumococcal strain and transformation protocol.
2. Plasmid for integration of constitutively expressed *lacI*: pPEPY-PF6-lacI (Addgene #85589).
3. Plasmid for integration of IPTG-inducible *dcas9*: pJWV102-PL-dCas9 (Addgene #85588).
4. C+Y medium [9, 10]
   (a) C+Y medium contains (total 110 mL): 100 mL PreC, 2.5 mL Adams III, 2.5 mL 10% yeast extract, 1 mL 8% BSA, 1.5 mL 2% sodium pyruvate, 1 mL 20% glucose, 0.5 mL 2 mg/mL uridine, 0.5 mL 2 mg/mL adenosine, 0.1 mL 0.4 mM $MnCl_2$, 0.073 mL 3% glutamine, 0.327 mL 0.3 M sucrose pH can be adjusted with HCl.
   (b) PreC contains 8.5 g/L K_2HPO_4, 5 g/L casein hydrolysate, 2 g/L sodium acetate, 11.25 mg/L cysteine, 6 mg/mL tryptophan.
   (c) Adams III contains 24 mg/L biotin, 24 mg/L nicotinic acid, 28 mg/L pyridoxine hydrochloride, 96 mg/L calcium pantothenate, 26 mg/L thiamine hydrochloride, 11 mg/L riboflavin, 20 mg/L $FeSO_4{\cdot}7H_2O$, 20 mg/L $CuSO_4{\cdot}5H_2O$, 20 mg/L $ZnSO_4{\cdot}7H_2O$, 8 mg/L $MnCl_2{\cdot}4H_2O$, 20 g/L $MgCl_2{\cdot}6H_2O$, 1.75 g/L L-asparagine, 200 mg/L choline, 0.5 g/L $CaCl_2$.
5. Todd Hewitt agar plates (Todd Hewitt broth supplemented with 1.5% agar) with 40 μg/mL gentamycin, 1 μg/mL tetracycline, or 100 μg/mL spectinomycin (*see* **Note 2**).
6. Isopropyl β-D-1-thiogalactopyranoside (IPTG).

3 Methods

3.1 Design and Construction of New sgRNAs for CRISPRi

The sgRNA construct consists of a 20 nt base-pairing region, a Cas9 handle and transcriptional terminator (Fig. 1). The latter two remain constant for all sgRNA constructs, while the base-pairing region ensures the gene specificity. When designing a novel sgRNA to target a gene of interest, there are several important criteria which needs to be taken into consideration:

1. The 20 nt base-pairing region should preferable bind to the nontemplate DNA strand close to the 5′ end of the gene or the

promoter region to obtain optimal efficiency. Binding to the template DNA strand has been shown to be less efficient [1].

2. The base-pairing region needs to be located adjacent to the protospacer adjacent motif (PAM) sequence of Cas9 [2]. The constructs designed by Liu et al. [3] utilize Cas9 from *Streptococcus pyogenes*, which has a 5′-NGG-3′ (any nucleotide followed by two guanosine nucleotides) PAM-sequence [6]. Partial targeting has also been observed for PAM-site 5′-NAG-3′ [7]. Only sequences next to 5′-NGG-3′ should be selected as base-pairing regions.
3. To ensure specific knockdown of the gene of interest, it is critical to ensure that the sgRNA does not target other genes in the genome. The 12 nts proximal to the PAM sequence (and thus the Cas9-handle in the sgRNA sequence) are most important for specificity. This sequence is known as the "seed sequence," and 1–2 differences here will dramatically reduce the binding efficiency of the sgRNA [1, 11]. BLAST searches should be performed to ensure that there are no off-target binding sites.
4. The secondary structure of the sgRNA needs to be intact for dCas9 to bind to the sgRNA-DNA complex. The folding of a newly designed sgRNA should therefore be checked using a secondary structure folding algorithm such as RNAfold from the ViennaRNA package [12] (http://rna.tbi.univie.ac.at/cgi-bin/RNAWebSuite/RNAfold.cgi) and compared to a functionally verified sgRNA.

As an example, I explain here how to design and construct an sgRNA plasmid targeting pneumococcal *pbp2a* gene (SPV_1821, SPD_1821, spr1823), encoding a bifunctional penicillin binding protein [13, 14], using inverse PCR (*see* **Note 3**).

1. Search the transcribed sequence (nontemplate strand) of the *pbp2a* gene (Fig. 1) for PAM-sequences 5′-CCN-3′ (reverse complement to 5′-NGG-3′ on the template strand). The 20 nt downstream of this PAM is a potential base-pairing sequence (Fig. 1) (*see* **Note 4**).
2. Perform a BLAST search against the full genome using the PAM-proximal 12 bp (seed sequence) as query. Discard any sgRNA whose seed sequence maps to a secondary site in the genome next to a PAM sequence.
3. Design the gene-specific primer for inverse PCR by adding the reverse complement of the 20 nt base-pairing sequence from the nontemplate strand to the annealing part of the forward primer (5′-GTTTAAGAGCTATGCTGGAAACAGC-3′). The resulting, gene-specific primer for *pbp2a* will thus be: 5′-<u>TTTTCGAATCGGACCTACTT</u>GTTTAAGAGCTATGCT

GGAAACAGC-3′ (base-pairing sequence is underlined) (Fig. 1).

4. To ensure that the secondary structure of the full sgRNA is not influenced by the base-pairing sequence, compare the secondary structure prediction of the new full sgRNA sequence (base-pairing region + Cas9 handle + transcriptional terminator (i.e., sgRNA(pbp2a); ATTTTCGAATCGGACCTACTTGTTTAAGAGCTATGCTGGAAACAGCATAGCAAGTTTAAATAAGGCTAGTCCGTTATCAACTTGAAAAAGTGGCACCGAGTCGGTGCTTTTTTTGAAGCTTGGGCCCGAACAAAAACTCAT) with that of a functionally verified sgRNA (e.g., sgRNA(luc); ATAGAGGATAGAATGGCGCCGTTTAAGAGCTATGCTGGAAACAGCATAGCAAGTTTAAATAAGGCTAGTCCGTTATCAACTTGAAAAAGTGGCACCGAGTCGGTGCTTTTTTTGAAGCTTGGGCCCGAACAAAAACTCAT) using RNAfold from the ViennaRNA package (http://rna.tbi.univie.ac.at/cgi-bin/RNAWebSuite/RNAfold.cgi) [12].
5. Order the verified oligo for inverse PCR.
6. Amplify new sgRNA vector using the following reaction:

	Volume (μL)
Phusion polymerase	0.5
HF buffer (10×)	10
dNTPs (2.5 mM each)	4
Universal primer (100 μM)	0.25
Specific primer (100 μM)	0.25
Template plasmid (100 ng/μL)	0.5
dH_2O	34.5
Total	50

The following cycling conditions are used:

Temperature (°C)	Time	
98	60 s	Initial denaturation
98 60 72	20 s 30 s 30 s/kbp	25 cycles
72	10 min	Final elongation

7. Cast a 1% agarose gel and perform electrophoresis. Purify the PCR product from gel using a PCR purification kit. Elute the

purified product PCR product in 20–30 μL elution buffer from the purification kit.

8. Set up two identical DpnI digestion reactions, to degrade template DNA (*see* **Note 5**).

	Volume (μL)
Purified PCR product	1
DpnI	1
Buffer (10×)	2
dH_2O	16
Total	20

Incubate the reaction at 37 °C for 2 h.

9. To circularize the plasmid, set up ligation reactions with the DpnI-digested PCR reactions without further purification. Include an extra reaction without ligase as a control.

	Inverse PCR reaction (volume in μL)	Control reaction (volume in μL)
Digestion mix	10	10
Ligase buffer (10×)	2	2
T4 DNA ligase	1	0
dH_2O	7	8
Total	20	20

Incubate at room temperature for 2 h or at 16 °C overnight.

10. Transform both ligation reactions to *E. coli* using conventional heat-shock procedures [15]. Plate out on LA plates containing 100 μg/mL spectinomycin for selection and incubate at 37 °C overnight.
11. The number of colonies of the plate with circularized plasmid should far exceed the number of colonies on the control plates (*see* **Note 6**). Pick a colony in LB with 100 μg/mL ampicillin and grow up 12–18 h.
12. Store the strain as freeze stock and isolate plasmid. Verify correct sgRNA by Sanger sequencing using sequencing primer (Ppepx_Seq_R; 5′-CGAGGGATTTGGTGATTCTTCTT-3′).

3.2 CRISPRi Strain Construction

The CRISPRi system developed by Liu et al. [3] relies on LacI-based IPTG-inducible expression of dCas9. In addition to the *dcas9* and sgRNA constructs, a *lacI* gene thus needs to be integrated into the chromosome of a strain to be used for CRISPRi. All constructs are available on plasmids via Addgene, and they all integrate into nonessential chromosomal loci by double crossover (*see* **Note 7**).

1. To introduce a constitutively expressed *lacI* into the pneumococcal genome, transform the plasmid pPEPY-PF6-*lacI* into the pneumococcal strain. The PF6-*lacI* construct will integrate into the *prs1* locus [3, 16, 17]. Select correct transformants by plating out on TH plates containing 40 μg/mL gentamycin.
2. Pick colonies in C+Y medium containing 40 μg/mL gentamycin (*see* **Note 8**) and grow until $OD_{600} = 0.4$ before the culture is stored as freeze stocks. Verify correct integration by PCR.
3. Next, transform the strain with plasmid pJWV102-PL-dCas9 [3], which integrates the LacI-dependent P_{lac}-*dcas9* construct into the *bgaA*-locus. Select transformants on TH plates with 1 μg/mL tetracycline.
4. Pick colonies in C+Y medium containing 1 μg/mL tetracycline (*see* **Note 8**) and grow until $OD_{600} = 0.4$ before the cultures are stored as freeze stocks. Verify correct integration by PCR. The resulting strain, carrying both constitutive *lacI* and IPTG-inducible *dcas9*, can be used to introduce different sgRNAs.
5. Finally, transform the strain with the constructed sgRNA plasmid (pPEPX-sgRNA). The constitutively expressed sgRNA will integrate into the region between the genes *amiF* and *treR*. Transformants are selected on TH agar plates with 100 μg/mL spectinomycin.
6. Pick colonies in C+Y medium containing 100 μg/mL spectinomycin (*see* **Note 8**) and grow until $OD_{600} = 0.4$ before the cultures are stored as freeze stocks. Verify correct integration by PCR.
7. The resulting strain is ready for CRISPRi knockdown experiment using an assay of choice. For example, grow the CRISPRi strain in C+Y medium without antibiotics until $OD_{600} = 0.4$. Then, dilute the culture in C+Y medium with 1 mM IPTG for maximum knockdown (*see* **Note 9**).

4 Notes

1. Phosphorylated primer can be ordered directly from oligo providers.
2. Columbia blood agar or other media are also possible to use. When plating pneumococci on top of the agar, the plates need to be incubated in anaerobic environment (anaerobic jars or 5% CO_2 incubators).
3. It is here described how to use inverse PCR to create new sgRNA plasmids (introduce new 20 bp sequences in the

vector). In addition to inverse PCR, Liu et al. [3] describes how to use infusion cloning for this purpose.

4. Automatic searches for base-pairing sequences can also be done using available software programs, such as CRISPR Primer Designer [18].
5. One of the parallel reactions will be used as negative control in the ligation reaction.
6. A large number of colonies on the control plate suggests that the DpnI reaction, which should degrade the template plasmids, has not worked properly. The DpnI treatment then needs to be repeated.
7. All vectors of the CRISPRi system constructed by Liu et al. [3] contain sequences with homology to the chromosome of *S. pneumoniae* D39, which allows them to integrate into nonessential chromosomal loci by double crossover. For utilization in other pneumococcal strains, the sequences of the homology regions should be similar to D39, and this should be checked before starting the experiment.
8. Instead of picking and growing the colonies in liquid medium containing antibiotics, the colonies can also be replated on antibiotic plates and incubated overnight. Replated colonies can then be picked and grown in liquid medium without antibiotics.
9. The CRISPRi system is titratable, and the level of knockdown can be adjusted by reducing the IPTG concentrations [3].

References

1. Qi LS, Larson MH, Gilbert LA, Doudna JA, Weissman JS, Arkin AP, Lim WA (2013) Repurposing CRISPR as an RNA-guided platform for sequence-specific control of gene expression. Cell 152:1173–1183
2. Jinek M, Chylinski K, Fonfara I, Hauer M, Doudna JA, Charpentier E (2012) A programmable dual-RNA-guided DNA endonuclease in adaptive bacterial immunity. Science 337:816–821
3. Liu X, Gallay C, Kjos M, Domenech A, Slager J, van Kessel SP, Knoops K, Sorg RA, Zhang JR, Veening JW (2017) High-throughput CRISPRi phenotyping identifies new essential genes in *Streptococcus pneumoniae*. Mol Syst Biol 13:931
4. Larson MH, Gilbert LA, Wang X, Lim WA, Weissman JS, Qi LS (2013) CRISPR interference (CRISPRi) for sequence-specific control of gene expression. Nat Protoc 8:2180–2196
5. Peters JM, Colavin A, Shi H, Czarny TL, Larson MH, Wong S, Hawkins JS, Lu CH, Koo BM, Marta E et al (2016) A comprehensive, CRISPR-based functional analysis of essential genes in bacteria. Cell 165:1493–1506
6. Bikard D, Jiang W, Samai P, Hochschild A, Zhang F, Marraffini LA (2013) Programmable repression and activation of bacterial gene expression using an engineered CRISPR-Cas system. Nucleic Acids Res 41:7429–7437
7. Jiang W, Bikard D, Cox D, Zhang F, Marraffini LA (2013) RNA-guided editing of bacterial genomes using CRISPR-Cas systems. Nat Biotechnol 31:233–239
8. van Raaphorst R, Kjos M, Veening JW (2017) Chromosome segregation drives division site selection in *Streptococcus pneumoniae*. Proc Natl Acad Sci U S A 114:E5959–E5968
9. Martin B, Garcia P, Castanie MP, Claverys JP (1995) The *recA* gene of *Streptococcus*

pneumoniae is part of a competence-induced operon and controls lysogenic induction. Mol Microbiol 15:367–379

10. Lacks S, Hotchkiss RD (1960) A study of the genetic material determining an enzyme in pneumococcus. Biochim Biophys Acta 39:508–518
11. Hawkins JS, Wong S, Peters JM, Almeida R, Qi LS (2015) Targeted transcriptional repression in bacteria using CRISPR interference (CRISPRi). Methods Mol Biol 1311:349–362
12. Lorenz R, Bernhart SH, Honer Zu Siederdissen C, Tafer H, Flamm C, Stadler PF, Hofacker IL (2011) ViennaRNA Package 2.0. Algorithms Mol Biol 6:26
13. Paik J, Kern I, Lurz R, Hakenbeck R (1999) Mutational analysis of the *Streptococcus pneumoniae* bimodular class A penicillin-binding proteins. J Bacteriol 181:3852–3856
14. Hoskins J, Matsushima P, Mullen DL, Tang J, Zhao G, Meier TI, Nicas TI, Jaskunas SR (1999) Gene disruption studies of penicillin-binding proteins 1a, 1b, and 2a in *Streptococcus pneumoniae*. J Bacteriol 181:6552–6555
15. Sambrook JF, Russell DW (2001) Molecular cloning: a laboratory manual, vol 1,2 and 3, 3rd edn. Cold Spring Harbor Laboratory Press, Cold Spring Harbor
16. Sorg RA, Kuipers OP, Veening JW (2015) Gene expression platform for synthetic biology in the human pathogen *Streptococcus pneumoniae*. ACS Synth Biol 4:228–239
17. Sorg RA (2016) Engineering approaches to investigate pneumococcal gene expression regulation and antibiotic resistance development. Ph.D. thesis, University of Groningen
18. Yan M, Zhou SR, Xue HW (2015) CRISPR primer designer: design primers for knockout and chromosome imaging CRISPR-Cas system. J Integr Plant Biol 57:613–617

Part IV

The Proteome and Proteomics of *Streptococcus pneumoniae*

Chapter 9

Protein Expression Analysis by Western Blot and Protein–Protein Interactions

María Dolores Cima-Cabal, Fernando Vazquez, Juan R. de los Toyos, and María del Mar García-Suárez

Abstract

Western blot analysis is widely used for detecting protein expression, analysis of protein–protein interactions, and searching for new biomarkers. Also, it is a diagnostic tool used for detection of human diseases and microorganism infections.

Some *Streptococcus pneumoniae* proteins are important virulence factors and a few of them are diagnostic markers. Here, we describe the detection of two pneumococcal proteins, pneumolysin and PpmA, in human urine by using monoclonal and polyclonal antibodies.

Key words Western-blot, Pneumolysin, PpmA, Monoclonal antibody, Urine

1 Introduction

The Western blot (WB) technique uses antibodies to identify target proteins via antigen–antibody specific reactions [1–3]. This technique remains as a rapid, simple, and cost-effective method for analysis of proteins. Firstly, a protein pool should be run on a sodium dodecyl sulfate–polyacrylamide gel electrophoresis (SDS-PAGE). Negatively charged and denaturalized proteins by SDS are separated into gel matrix in function of their molecular weight, followed by their electrophoretic transfer onto a nitrocellulose o PVDF sheet [4–6].

Specific detection of protein targets is achieved by using monoclonal or polyclonal antibodies, and secondary antibody conjugates with horseradish peroxidase or alkaline phosphatase. Initially, immunochemically stained bands were obtained by using NBT and BICP, yielding highly colored, water-insoluble products. Increasing detection sensitivity was achieved by chemiluminescence reactions. Luminol reactions are preferred to detect picogram levels of protein in a sample [7].

Federico Iovino (ed.), *Streptococcus pneumoniae: Methods and Protocols*, Methods in Molecular Biology, vol. 1968, https://doi.org/10.1007/978-1-4939-9199-0_9,

On the other hand, the fluorescence detection method focused attention because it is more quantitative and is suitable for the detection of multiple proteins simultaneously, although is limited by low detection sensitivity [8, 9].

WB is also used to detect protein–protein interactions in vitro. The technique was a derivative of standard WB and named "Far western blot" [10]. Further fine description and applications of this technique are beyond the scope of this chapter.

WB is a tool for the diagnosis of various infections and diseases [11]. It is commonly used in the serodiagnosis of parasitic diseases as toxocariasis [12], echinococcosis [13, 14], toxoplasmosis [15], trichinellosis [16] and fungal diseases as aspergillosis [17, 18]. HIV serodiagnosis [19, 20] and borreliosis [21] use WB as a confirmatory step to guarantee positive identification.

Streptococcus pneumoniae causes serious invasive diseases, mainly pneumonia, meningitis, and bacteremia, in addition to otitis media and acute sinusitis. Pneumolysin (PLY) is a 53-kDa protein with biological activities implicated in virulence and the early stages of the biofilm formation process [22–26]. PLY belongs to the family of antigenically related thiol-activated, cholesterol-binding cytolysins, secreted by species of five genera of gram-positive bacteria [27–29].

On the other hand, the putative proteinase maturation protein A (PpmA) of *S. pneumoniae* is homologous to members of the family of peptidyl-prolyl cis–trans isomerases (PPIases), which accelerate the rate-limiting cis–trans or trans–cis conformational changes at X-Pro bonds during protein folding. Some PPIases are involved in bacterial virulence [30, 31]. Pneumococcal PpmA is a 34.4-kDa lipoprotein which elicits protective immune responses and is involved in pneumococcal colonization [32, 33].

A key factor for prognosis in pneumonia is to recognize the underlying microorganisms and subsequently managing the appropriate antimicrobial chemotherapy [34].

Human urine is a noninvasive sample, easy to obtain, and relatively stable [35]. Human urine is, in fact, used to diagnose viral, bacterial, and fungal infections such as tuberculosis [36], *Helicobacter pylori* infection [37], leptospirosis [38], histoplasmosis [39], and dengue fever [40].

Here we describe the detection of antigenic proteins in human urine for the diagnosis of pneumococcal pneumonia using WB [41, 42].

2 Materials

2.1 Urine Samples: Collection and Preparation

Urine samples were obtained from patients with suspected community-acquired pneumonia admitted to three hospitals in Asturias, Spain (Hospital Universitario Central de Asturias, Hospital Monte Naranco, and Hospital San Agustín). Samples from healthy adults were obtained from volunteer subjects at the School of Medicine, and samples from healthy children were obtained during routine pediatric checkups at a health care center in Lugones (Asturias, Spain).

Samples were collected (100 ml sterile urine collection cup with integrated transfer device, and 100 ml sterile pediatric urine collection bag) upon admission or during the first day of hospitalization, and a solution with five protease inhibitors was added (1 to 20 volumes of sample) and frozen at −70 °C until use. The protease inhibitors solution was made up of 100 mM EDTA in distilled water, 100 mM N-ethyl-maleimide in ethanol, 100 mM PMSF in ethanol, pepstatin (100 μ/ml in PBS), and leupeptin (200 μg/ml in distilled water); the proportion of each component was 1:5 in the final volume.

2.2 Antigens and Antibodies

Recombinant PLY (1–10 ng) was used as control in WB PLY assay. PLY was expressed and purified as previously reported [43]. The total protein concentration was colorimetrically estimated applying the Bio-Rad (Bradford) protein assay. Recombinant PpmA was used as previously reported [42].

Monoclonal antibody PLY-7 and anti-PpmA hyperimmune rabbit serum were obtained as previously described [42, 44]. Peroxidase-conjugated goat anti-mouse IgG (whole molecule) can be commercially acquired.

2.3 SDS-PAGE Materials and Reagents

The following materials and reagents are necessary for electrophoretic separation of proteins by SDS–polyacrylamide gel electrophoresis (SDS-PAGE).

1. Bio-Rad minigel system (Bio-Rad Laboratories, Richmond, CA, USA).
2. *Sample buffer (4×)*: 200 mM Tris–HCl, pH 6.8, 400 mM DTT (DL-Dithiothreitol, Sigma-Aldrich), 0.1% Bromophenol Blue (BPB, Sigma-Aldrich), 8% SDS (Bio-Rad), 40% glycerol. Leave one aliquot at 4 °C for current use and store the remaining aliquots at −20 °C. *See* that SDS precipitates at 4 °C, so it is necessary to warm the sample buffer prior to use.
3. *SDS-PAGE running buffer*: Prepare a mixture of 3 g of Tris (Tris base, 2-amino-2-(hydroxymethyl)-1,3-propanediol), 14.4 g of glycine, and 1 g of SDS (sodium dodecyl sulfate; Bio-Rad) in 1 L of ultrapure water. Do not adjust the pH and store at room temperature.
4. *1.5 M Tris–HCl, pH 8.8*: Add about 100 ml ultrapure water to a 1 L graduated cylinder. Weigh 181.7 g Tris and transfer to the cylinder. Use a magnetic stir bar to allow that the Tris dissolves quickly into the water, then add water to a volume of 900 ml.

Mix and adjust pH with HCl (1 N). Make up to 1 L with ultrapure water and store at 4 °C.

5. *0.5 M Tris–HCl, pH 6.8*: Weigh 60.6 g Tris and prepare a 1 L solution as in previous step. Store at 4 °C.
6. *30% Acrylamide–Bis solution (30:0.8) acrylamide–bis-acrylamide*: Weigh 30 g of acrylamide monomer and 0.8 g bis-acrylamide (N,N′-methylenebis(acrylamide)) and transfer to an 100 ml graduated cylinder containing about 40 ml of water and mix for about 30 min. Make up to 100 ml with water and filter through a 0.45 μm filter. Store at 4 °C, in a bottle wrapped with aluminum foil, for 1 month. *See* that is important to wear a mask and gloves when weighing acrylamide to avoid exposition to this neurotoxin.

2.4 Western Blotting: Materials and Reagents

1. Bio-Rad mini Trans-Blot system (Bio-Rad Laboratories, Richmond, CA, USA).
2. Poly (vinylidene difluoride) membranes (PVDF) (Immobilon-P; Millipore, Bedford, MA, USA).
3. Whatman® 3 MM blotting paper.
4. BM Chemiluminescence Western Blotting Substrate (POD) (Roche).
5. Kodak Carestream® Kodak® BioMax® light film.
6. Kodak® exposure cassette.
7. Transfer buffer: Prepare a mixture of 3 g of Tris, 14.4 g of glycine, 200 ml of methanol, and 800 ml of ultrapure water.
8. Tris-buffered saline (TBS): dilute 6.05 g of Tris (50 mM) and 8.76 g of NaCl (150 mM) in 900 ml of distilled water and mix. Adjust pH at 7.5 with HCl (1 N) and make to 1 L with water.
9. TBS containing 0.05% Tween 20 (TBST): Separate 500 ml of TBS and add 250 μl of Tween 20; note that is important to cut the end of blue tip to aspirate Tween 20 easily.
10. Blocking buffer: 1% blocking reagent (Roche) in TBS is prepared the day before and store at 4 °C. This reagent is used for nucleic acid hybridization and detection; however, it provides an efficient blocking of PVDF membranes. On the other hand, it is hard to dissolve, even on a heating block.
11. Diluent antibody solution: 0.5% blocking reagent in TBS, prepared the same day or stored at 4 °C.
12. Ponceau S Staining Solution: 0.5 g Ponceau S in 1 ml acetic acid, complete with ultrapure water to 10 ml. Store at 4 °C. Do not freeze.

3 Methods

3.1 Urine Sample Preparation

Prior to analysis, the frozen samples are thawed out at room temperature overnight. The protease inhibitors solution aims to preserve the potential protein degradation during urine thawing (*see* **Note 1**).

20 ml of urine samples is spun at 3000 × *g* for 2 min, and the supernatant is removed. Triton X-100 is added to the samples a 0.1% final concentration and incubated at 37 °C for 30 min (*see* **Note 2**). Triton X-100 is added to the samples to minimize the interactions with other components of the urine, as previously observed [41].

After that, the samples are concentrated (about 20 times) using Vivaspin Turbo 15, 3000 MWCO PES (Sartorius). Concentrated proteins are recovered and stored at 4 °C or frozen until use (*see* **Note 3**).

3.2 SDS–Polyacrylamide Gel Electrophoresis

Cast the gel glasses of the Bio-Rad minigel system following the manufacturer's instructions. Prepare the gel mixtures for 12% SDS–polyacrylamide gels.

Running gel: Prepare a mixture of 3.5 ml of ultrapure water; 2.5 ml of 1.5 M Tris–HCl, pH 8.8; 100 μl of 10% SDS; 4 ml of 30%:0.8% acrylamide–bis solution; 50 μl of 10% ammonium persulfate; 5 μl of N,N,N′,N-tetramethylethylenediamine (TEMED, Sigma). Load gel glasses with 5 ml of the mix, and add 1 ml of water on top to allow the gel to polymerize with a levelled straight front line.

Stacking gel: Prepare a mixture of 6.1 ml of ultrapure water; 2.5 ml of 0.5 M Tris–HCl, pH 6.8; 100 μl of 10% SDS; 1.3 ml of 30%:0.8% acrylamide–bis solution; 50 μl of 10% ammonium persulfate; 5 μl of TEMED. Remove all water, load mix and insert the 10-well gel comb.

Urine samples (15 μl), protein controls (PLY and PpmA), and protein MW standards (Broad or low range protein MW, Bio-Rad) are mixed with sample buffer (4×), boiled for 5 min and centrifuged at 3000 × *g* for 30 s. (*see* **Note 4**). Thereafter, samples are loaded into the gels and separated by applying 120 V (20 mA) for 1.5–2 h, until the Bromophenol Blue front reaches the gel end (*see* **Note 5**).

3.3 Western Blotting

The proteins are then transferred to PVDF membranes (Immobilon-P), using a mini-trans-blot system.

For that, prepare pieces of PVDF membranes of a similar size to the mini gels, mark with a pencil the sample lanes, wet in methanol for a few seconds and transfer into a container with transfer buffer. Also, prepare pieces of Whatman® 3 MM blotting paper of similar size to the PVDF pieces and soak them in transfer buffer. For this process wear gloves and handle papers and membranes carefully using tweezers.

Carefully remove the gels from the glasses and submerge them in transfer buffer. Prepare the gel–membrane sandwich (*see* **Note 6**). Proceed following manufacturer's instructions. For protein transference, we usually apply 300 mA for 2 h (*see* **Note 7**).

When the transference is finished, the membranes are stained with Ponceau S for about 5 min at room temperature and gentle shaking until protein bands are visible. Mark protein bands with a pencil if you like. Add water for destaining for 2–10 min, until the stain is mostly removed. After that, rinse the membranes several times with TBS. Subsequently, the membranes are blocked in TBS containing 1% blocking reagent for 1 h at room temperature with gentle shaking or overnight at 4 °C (without shaking).

Before starting with the protein detection, place the BM Chemiluminescence Western Blotting Substrate (POD) at room temperature.

For WB PLY detection (Fig. 1): Monoclonal antibody PLY-7 is used at 10 μg/sample in diluent antibody solution and added to the membrane strips. Place the container in a rocking shaker with gentle agitation. After 1 h of incubation at room temperature, membrane strips are profusely washed three times (10 min each) with TBS–Tween 20 (0.05%). Additional wash with TBS containing 0.5% blocking reagent is done to eliminate all remaining Tween 20.

Goat anti-mouse IgG (whole molecule) peroxidase conjugate (diluted 1:2000) is added, and the strips are incubated for 30 min at room temperature.

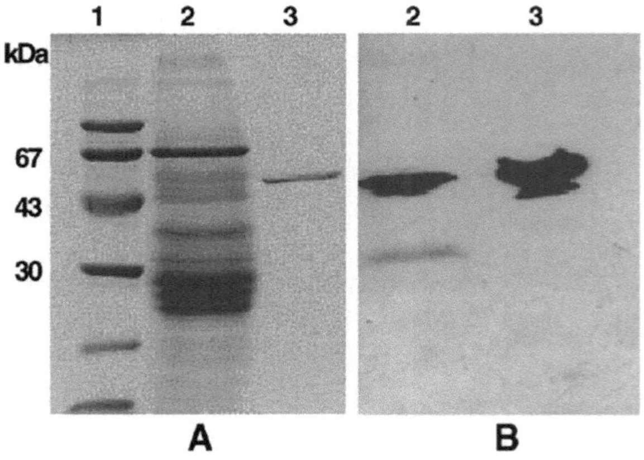

Fig. 1 Detection of pneumolysin in human urine. Coomassie Brilliant Blue-stained 12% gel SDS-PAGE (Panel **a**) and Western blot analysis with the mouse monoclonal antibody PLY-7 (Panel **b**) of the HCV 34 urine sample concentrate. Lane 1: molecular weight markers, lane 2: HCV 34 urine concentrate, lane 3: 1 μg of recombinant PLY in PBS (reproduced from ref. 41 with permission from Elsevier). HCV 34 is a sample from an adult patient

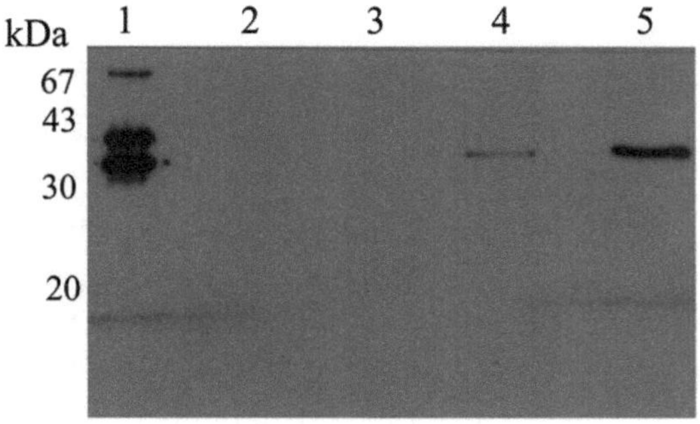

Fig. 2 Detection of proteinase maturation protein A (PpmA) in human urine by Western blot. Anti-PpmA hyperimmune rabbit serum was incubated with recombinant PpmA (lane 1), urine samples from healthy children (lanes 2 and 3), and urine samples from pediatric patients with pneumococcal pneumonia (lane 4 and 5). Low range protein MW are marked at left

For WB PpmA detection (Fig. 2): Anti-PpmA hyperimmune rabbit serum is diluted 1:1000 in diluent antibody solution and added to the membrane strips. Place the container in a rocking shaker with gentle agitation. Membrane strips are treated as above except that goat anti-rabbit IgG (whole molecule) peroxidase conjugate is diluted 1:5000.

During this step, prepare the detection solution by mixing solutions A and B using BM Chemiluminescence Western Blotting Substrate (POD), following manufacturer's instructions (*see* **Note 8**). Wrap the tube with aluminum foil and keep at room temperature. Place the rest of Chemiluminescence Western Blotting Substrate (POD) kit again at 4 °C. After washing four times (10 min each) with TBST, add TBS to the membranes and stop shaking. Prepare an exposition cassette by placing a piece of cellophane, enough to wrap the membrane. Take the exposition cassette, the Kodak film, the developing solution, a timer and a glass container and go to the dark room. Prepare the Kodak solutions for film development.

Drain carefully the membrane and place it into a container. Take care the protein side is in the upper face (*see* **Note 9**). Add the developing solution in the container and count for 1 min; shake very gently so that the solution is evenly distributed for all the membrane surface (*see* **Note 10**).

Drain as much as possible the membrane before placing over the cellophane. Take care not to leave bubbles between the cellophane and the PVDF membrane when wrapping with cellophane (*see* **Note 11**). Place a Kodak film and count for 1 min, making sure where the position of the membrane is (*see* **Notes 12** and **13**).

4 Notes

1. Urine samples could be defrosted at 4 °C, but it takes more time.
2. Urine samples often show salt precipitation during the freezing process. In addition, especially in the urine samples from patients, which show visible traces of blood and tissues, these need to be removed before running into SDS-PAGE.
3. Take off all filter adsorbed protein by applying small volume of PBS with 0.1% SDS.
4. Usually we prefer to make two identical gels, one for Coomassie Blue staining and the other one for electrotransference for WB detection (which is treated with Ponceau S Stain for WB in order to check that all the protein is electrotransferred).
5. If there are samples with potential high protein concentration, leave empty wells between samples. Because the high sensitivity of chemiluminescence detection, any tiny leak protein can easily confuse the results and lead to false positives.
6. Do not allow the membrane to dry out and avoid bubbles between gel and membrane.
7. Make sure that the ice container/cooling unit is not defrosted during the process in order to maintain protein transference at low temperature. To homogenize temperature in all the transfer buffer, we use a magnetic stir bar inside the transfer container and place it on a stirrer.
8. We use a 10 ml tube with 3 ml solution A (100 μl solution B) for each membrane corresponding to one gel.
9. The membrane protein side is the face in contact with the gel during electrophoretic transfer.
10. This step is crucial, and the developing solution must be in contact with every piece of membrane, even if more than 1 min is necessary to have the whole membrane submerged.
11. Remove any excess of liquid with a paper.
12. Cut a little piece of the film to identify the lane positions, for example, the bottom corner on the left, before placing onto the cassette.
13. If you do not know the expected intensity of signal, place successively several Kodak films with 1 min, 5 min, 10 min, etc. of exposition time.

Acknowledgments

The authors acknowledge Dr. Federico Iovino from Karolinska Institute for inviting us to write this chapter and for reviewing the manuscript, and Dr. Fermín Torrano for his constant support in the preparation of this chapter.

References

1. Towbin H, Staehelin T, Gordon J (1979) Electrophoretic transfer of proteins from polyacrylamide gels to nitrocellulose sheets: procedure and some applications. Proc Natl Acad Sci U S A 76:4350–4354
2. Magi B, Liberatori S (2005) Immunoblotting techniques. Methods Mol Biol 295:227–254
3. Chi-Chih K, Yamauchi KA, Vlassakis J, Sinkala E, Duncombe TA, Herr AE (2016) Single cell-resolution western blotting. Nat Protoc 11:1508–1530
4. Burnette WN (1981) "Western blotting": electrophoretic transfer of proteins from sodium dodecyl sulfate-polyacrylamide gels to unmodified nitrocellulose and radiographic detection with antibody and radioiodinated protein A. Anal Biochem 112:195–203
5. Pluskal M, Przekop M, Kavonian M (1986) Immobilon® PVDF transfer membrane: a new membrane substrate for Western blotting of proteins. BioTechniques 4:272–283
6. Komatsu S (2015) Western blotting using PVDF membranes and its downstream applications. Methods Mol Biol 1312:227–236
7. Yakunin AF, Hallenbeck PC (2001) A luminol/iodophenol chemiluminescent detection system for western immunoblots. In: Van Dyke K, Van Dyke C, Woodfork K (eds) Luminescence biotechnology: instruments and applications. CRC Press
8. Gingrich JC, Davis DR, Nguyen Q (2000) Multiplex detection and quantitation of proteins on western blots using fluorescent probes. BioTechniques 29:636–642
9. Kondo Y, Higa S, Iwasaki T, Matsumoto T, Maehara K, Harada A, Baba Y, Fujita M, Ohkawa Y (2018) Sensitive detection of fluorescence in western blotting by merging images. PLoS One 13:e0191532
10. Wu Y, Li Q, Chen XZ (2007) Detecting protein-protein interactions by far western blotting. Nat Protoc 2:3278–3284
11. Rognon B, Reboux G, Roussel S, Barrera C, Dalphin JC, Fellrath JM, Monod M, Millon L (2015) Western blotting as a tool for the serodiagnosis of farmer's lung disease: validation with *Lichtheimia corymbifera* protein extracts. J Med Microbiol 64:359–368
12. García HH, Cancrini G, Bartalesi F, Rodriguez S, Jimenez JA, Roldan W, Mantella A, Nicoletti A, Bartoloni A (2007) Evaluation of immunodiagnostics for toxocarosis in experimental porcine cysticercosis. Tropical Med Int Health 12:107–110
13. Tappe D, Grüner B, Kern P, Frosch M (2008) Evaluation of a commercial *Echinococcus* Western blot assay for serological follow-up of patients with alveolar echinococcosis. Clin Vaccine Immunol 15:1633–1637
14. Aslan M, Yüksel P, Polat E, Cakan H, Ergin S, Öner YA, Zengin K, Arıkan S, Saribas S, Torun MM, Kocazeybek B (2011) The diagnostic value of Western blot method in patients with cystic echinococcosis. New Microbiol 34:173–177
15. Magi B, Migliorini L (2011) Western blotting for the diagnosis of congenital toxoplasmosis. New Microbiol 34:93–95
16. Gómez-Morales MA, Ludovisi A, Amati M, Blaga R, Zivojinovic M, Ribicich M, Pozio E (2012) A distinctive Western blot pattern to recognize *Trichinella* infections in humans and pigs. Int J Parasitol 42:1017–1023
17. Madan T, Priyadarsiny P, Vaid M, Kamal N, Shah A, Haq W, Katti SB, Sarma PU (2004) Use of a synthetic peptide epitope of asp f 1, a major allergen or antigen of *Aspergillus fumigatus*, for improved immunodiagnosis of allergic bronchopulmonary aspergillosis. Clin Diagn Lab Immunol 11:552–558
18. Stopiglia CDO, Arechavala A, Carissimi M, Sorrentino JM, Aquino VR, Daboit TC, Kammler L, Negroni R, Scroferneker ML (2012) Standardization and characterization of antigens for the diagnosis of aspergillosis. Can J Microbiol 58:455–462
19. Torian LV, Forgione LA, Punsalang AE, Pirillo RE, Oleszko WR (2011) Comparison of multispot EIA with Western blot for confirmatory serodiagnosis of HIV. J Clin Virol 52:S41–S44

20. Hughesa AJ, Herra AE (2012) Microfluidic Western blotting. Proc Natl Acad Sci U S A 109:21450–21455
21. Evans R, Mavin S, McDonagh S, Chatterton JM, Milner R, Ho-Yen DO (2010) More specific bands in the IgG western blot in sera from Scottish patients with suspected Lyme borreliosis. J Clin Pathol 63:719–721
22. Gilbert RJ, Jiménez JL, Chen S, Tickle IJ, Rossjohn J, Parker M, Andrew PW, Saibil HR (1999) Two structural transitions in membrane pore formation by pneumolysin, the pore-forming toxin of *Streptococcus pneumoniae*. Cell 97:647–655
23. Coleman JR, Papamichail D, Yano M, García-Suárez MM, Pirofski LA (2011) Designed reduction of *Streptococcus pneumoniae* pathogenicity via synthetic changes in virulence factor codon-pair bias. J Infect Dis 203:1264–1273
24. Shak JR, Ludewick HP, Howery KE, Sakai F, Yi H, Harvey RM, Paton JC, Klugman KP, Vidal JE (2013) Novel role for the *Streptococcus pneumoniae* toxin pneumolysin in the assembly of biofilms. MBio 4:e00655–e00613. https://doi.org/10.1128/mBio.00655-13.
25. Mitchell TJ, Dalziel CE (2014) The biology of pneumolysin. Subcell Biochem 80:145–160
26. Khan MN, Coleman JR, Vernatter J, Varshney AK, Dufaud C, Pirofski LA (2014) An ahemolytic pneumolysin of *Streptococcus pneumoniae* manipulates human innate and CD4$^+$ T-cell responses and reduces resistance to colonization in mice in a serotype-independent manner. J Infect Dis 210:1658–1669
27. Gilbert RJ (2010) Cholesterol-dependent cytolysins. Adv Exp Med Biol 677:56–66
28. Farrand AJ, Hotze EM, Sato TK, Wade KR, Wimley WC, Johnson AE, Tweten RK (2015) The cholesterol-dependent cytolysin membrane-binding interface discriminates lipid environments of cholesterol to support β-barrel pore insertion. J Biol Chem 290:17733–17744
29. Lukoyanova N, Hoogenboom BW, Saibil HR (2016) The membrane attack complex, perforin and cholesterol-dependent cytolysin superfamily of pore-forming proteins. J Cell Sci 129:2125–2133
30. Ünal CM, Steinert M (2014) Microbial peptidyl-prolyl cis/trans isomerases (PPIases): virulence factors and potential alternative drug targets. Microbiol Mol Biol Rev 78:544–571
31. Dimou M, Venieraki A, Katinakis P (2017) Microbial cyclophilins: specialized functions in virulence and beyond. World J Microbiol Biotechnol 33:164. https://doi.org/10.1007/s11274-017-2330-6
32. Overweg K, Kerr A, Sluijter M, Jackson MH, Mitchell TJ, de Jong AP, de Groot R, Hermans PW (2000) The putative proteinase maturation protein A of *Streptococcus pneumoniae* is a conserved surface protein with potential to elicit protective immune responses. Infect Immun 7:4180–4188
33. Hermans PW, Adrian PV, Albert C, Estevão S, Hoogenboezem T, Luijendijk IH, Kamphausen T, Hammerschmidt S (2006) The streptococcal lipoprotein rotamase A (SlrA) is a functional peptidyl-prolyl isomerase involved in pneumococcal colonization. J Biol Chem 281:968–976
34. Cilloniz C, Martin-Loeches I, Garcia-Vidal C, San Jose A, Torres A (2016) Microbial etiology of pneumonia: epidemiology, diagnosis and resistance patterns. Int J Mol Sci 17:2120. https://doi.org/10.3390/ijms17122120
35. Saukkoriipi A, Pascal T, Palmu AA (2016) Evaluation of the BinaxNOW® *Streptococcus pneumoniae* antigen test on fresh, frozen and concentrated urine samples in elderly patients with and without community-acquired pneumonia. J Microbiol Methods 121:24–26
36. Gina P, Randall PJ, Muchinga TE, Pooran A, Meldau R, Peter JG, Dheda K (2017) Early morning urine collection to improve urinary lateral flow LAM assay sensitivity in hospitalised patients with HIV-TB co-infection. BMC Infect Dis 17:339. https://doi.org/10.1186/s12879-017-2313-0
37. Syam AF, Miftahussurur M, Uwan W, Simanjuntak D, Uchida T, Yamaoka Y (2015) Validation of urine test for detection of *Helicobacter pylori* infection in Indonesian population. Biomed Res Int 2015:152823. https://doi.org/10.1155/2015/152823
38. Saengjaruk P, Chaicumpa W, Watt G, Bunyaraksyotin G, Wuthiekanun V, Tapchaisri P, Sittinont C, Panaphut T, Tomanakan K, Sakolvaree Y, Chongsa-Nguan-M, Mahakunkijcharoen Y, Kalambaheti T, Naigowit P, Wambangco MAL, Kurazono H, Hayashi H (2002) Diagnosis of human leptospirosis by monoclonal antibody-based antigen detection in urine. J Clin Microbiol 40:480–489
39. Theel ES, Jespersen DJ, Harring J, Mandrekar J, Binnicker MJ (2013) Evaluation of an enzyme immunoassay for detection of histoplasma capsulatum antigen from urine specimens. J Clin Microbiol 51:3555–3559
40. Chuansumrit A, Chaiyaratana W, Tangnararatchakit K, Yoksan S, Flamand M, Sakuntabhai A (2011) Dengue nonstructural protein 1 antigen in the urine as a rapid and convenient diagnostic test during the febrile

stage in patients with dengue infection. Diagn Microbiol Infect Dis 71:467–469

41. Cima-Cabal MD, Méndez FJ, Vázquez F, Aranaz C, Rodríguez-Alvarez J, García-García JM, Fleites A, Martínez González-Río J, Molinos L, de Miguel D, de los Toyos JR (2003) Immunodetection of pneumolysin in human urine by ELISA. J Microbiol Methods 54:47–55
42. García-Suárez MM, Cron LE, Suárez-Alvarez B, Villaverde R, González-Rodríguez I, Vázquez F, Hermans PW, Méndez FJ (2009) Diagnostic detection of *Streptococcus pneumoniae* PpmA in urine. Clin Microbiol Infect 15:443–453
43. Cima-Cabal MD, Vázquez F, de los Toyos JR, Méndez FJ (1999) Rapid and reliable identification of *Streptococcus pneumoniae* isolates by pneumolysin-mediated agglutination. J Clin Microbiol 37:1964–1966
44. de los Toyos JR, Mendez FJ, Aparicio JF, Vazquez F, Garcia-Suarez MM, Fleites A, Hardisson C, Morgan PJ, Andrew PW, Mitchell TJ (1996) Functional analysis of pneumolysin by use of monoclonal antibodies. Infect Immun 64:480–484

Chapter 10

Mass Spectrometry to Study the Bacterial Proteome from a Single Colony

Jianwei Zhou, Lu Zhang, Huixia Chuan, Angela Sloan, Raymond Tsang, and Keding Cheng

Abstract

Mass spectrometry (MS) has been widely used in recent years for bacterial identification and typing. Single bacterial colonies are regarded as pure cultures of bacteria grown from single cells. In this chapter, we describe a method for identifying bacteria at the species level with 100% accuracy using the proteomes of bacterial cultures from single colonies. In this chapter, six reference strains of gram-negative and gram-positive bacteria are analyzed, producing results of high reproducibility, as examples of bacterial identification through the application of liquid chromatography–tandem mass spectrometry (LC-MS/MS) and a custom database. Details on sample preparation and identification of *Streptococcus pneumoniae* are also described.

Key words Bacterial identification, Mass spectrometry, *Streptococcus pneumoniae*, LC-MS/MS, Single colonies

1 Introduction

Mass spectrometry (MS), especially matrix-assisted laser desorption/ionization time-of-flight (MALDI-TOF) MS, has been widely used for bacterial identification. Current MALDI-TOF MS platforms can identify bacteria at the genus, species, and subspecies levels, with different bacteria showing various accuracies at different levels [1]. We have used both liquid chromatography–tandem mass spectrometry (LC-MS/MS) and MALDI-TOF MS in the past few years to identify and type bacteria at the subspecies level [2–4]. Although MALDI-TOF MS is very fast for bacterial identification, it needs special sample preparation to enrich the molecules of interest and sometimes repeated sample runs are required to reach bacterial identification at the subspecies level [3, 4]. In MS-based bacterial identification and typing, accurate databases also play an important role in obtaining accurate results [1].

Federico Iovino (ed.), *Streptococcus pneumoniae: Methods and Protocols*, Methods in Molecular Biology, vol. 1968, https://doi.org/10.1007/978-1-4939-9199-0_10,

In this chapter, we introduce an easy and accurate method for identifying bacteria from single colonies at the species level using the LC-MS/MS approach. We feel that this method will play a practical role in identifying different bacteria in laboratories performing routine bacterial identification.

2 Materials

Prepare all solutions with ultrapure water (conductivity measured to 18.2 mΩ).

2.1 Bacteria Culture

1. 10 μl culture loops.
2. 100 × 15 mm trypticase soy agar (TSA) culture plates with 5% sheep blood:
   4% trypticase soy agar, 95% (v/v) H_2O, 5% (v/v) sheep blood.
3. 100 × 15 mm Columbia culture plates with 5% sheep blood:
   4.3% Columbia blood agar base, 95% H_2O, 5% (v/v) sheep blood.
4. 1.5 ml low-retention microcentrifuge tubes.
5. 25G needle.
6. 1 ml syringe.
7. 1 ml pipette tips, long (Thermo Scientific).

2.2 Tryptic Digestion

Prepare all solutions with ultrapure water (conductivity measured to 18.2 mΩ) and LC/MS-grade reagents.

1. 100 mM ammonium bicarbonate: add 0.4 mg ammonium bicarbonate (AB; Sigma) to 50 ml water.
2. 10% formic acid: Dilute 99.5+% formic acid 1:10 with water (FA; Fisher Canada).
3. Spin filters with a 30 kD molecular weight (MW) cutoff (Millipore).
4. Trypsin solution: dissolve 100 μg trypsin (Promega or Pierce, ThermoFisher) into 1.0 ml 100 mM AB immediately before use.

2.3 LC-MS/MS Runs

1. 0.3 × 5 mm C18 precolumn (ThermoFisher).
2. LTQ-Orbitrap XL system (ThermoFisher).
3. Mascot 2.3 (Matrix Science) software.
4. Bacteria GID database. (The author's institute can supply if requested.)

3 Methods

Carry out all procedures at room temperature, unless otherwise noted. In keeping with aseptic techniques, a biological safety cabinet should be used to perform any procedure involving bacteria.

3.1 Bacterial Culture

1. Streak gram-negative bacteria onto TSA containing 5% sheep blood and culture overnight at 37 °C.
2. Culture gram-positive bacteria on Columbia agar containing 5% sheep blood and 5% carbon dioxide at 37 °C overnight or until colonies are observed.
3. When spreading the bacterial cells on the plate, ensure that several substreaks are made so that single colonies can be obtained. Different cells have different growth rates and colony shapes.
4. Special attention should be paid to *Streptococcus pneumoniae*, which may grow slower than the other bacteria mentioned here. Further, the colony centers of these bacteria are normally found depressed when cultured for longer than 24 h.

3.2 Picking Colonies

1. Long 1 ml pipette tips are of suitable length for picking colonies. Place the tip close to parallel to the surface of the culture plate. Touch, wipe, and then turn the tip so that the maximum amount of colony can be lifted.
2. For *Streptococcus pneumoniae* colonies with depressed centers, use a 25G needle to make a shallow cut on the semisolid agar along the perimeter of the colony first, and then make a thin cut underneath the colony with the needle. The colony along with the thin layer of agar can then be picked up by pricking and lifting the agar with the needle and putting into the centrifuge tube.
3. Dip the end of the tip into a 1.5 ml low-retention microcentrifuge tube containing 50 μl of water, making several turns to guarantee the content of the colony is released into the water. Depress the pipette plunger in order to discharge any liquid out of the tip.
4. For *Streptococcus pneumoniae* colony along with the thin layer of agar, the agar piece is directly put into the centrifuge tube by the needle.

3.3 Tryptic Digestion

1. Quickly vortex the single colony cultures at low speed to ensure that the bacteria are fully suspended.
2. Remove a vial of trypsin (100 μg/vial, *see* **Note 1**) from the freezer and add 100 mM AB so that the final trypsin concentration is 100 ng/μl. Quickly vortex.

3. Add 50 μl trypsin solution to each sample.
4. Allow the digestion to proceed at 37 °C for at least 1 h (*see* **Note 2**).

3.4 Preparation of Samples for LC-MS/MS

1. Quickly spin down each sample and transfer the supernatant (approximately 100 μl) onto a 30 kDa MW cutoff spin column filter equilibrated with 10 μl 1% FA (*see* **Note 3**).
2. Centrifuge the spin column for 10 min at 10,000 × *g* and collect the filtrate.
3. Submit each sample for LC-MS/MS analysis.

3.5 LC-MS/MS and Database Search

1. Load 10 μl of each sample, representing one-tenth of the tryptic digest, onto a 0.3 × 5 mm C18 precolumn and let the sample bind to the precolumn for 6 min, then let the precolumn connected to a self-packed C18 nano-LC column. (The software can make them automatically connected.)
2. Run the Nano-LC (Proxeon) separation at 300 nl/min with a 45 min acetonitrile gradient from 5 to 36% followed by a 5 min flush with 95% acetonitrile and 10 min equilibration with buffer A.
3. When running multiple samples, perform two blank runs: (1) the first (termed "jigsaw") to wash the nanocolumn vigorously with several cycles of high concentration acetonitrile, and (2) the second using the same gradient used to run true samples to reflush and equilibrate the column for the next sample [4] (*see* **Note 4**).
4. Collect MS data from an LTQ-Orbitrap XL system with a data-dependent acquisition method for peptide ion scanning and fragmentation.
5. Search the MS data against a custom general identification database (GID) using Mascot 2.3. Use search parameters of 30 ppm mass error tolerance and two missed cleavages of trypsin digestion with no fixed modifications of proteins and possible modifications of methionine oxidation. Use the top hit in the database search list as the bacterial identification hit (*see* Fig. 1 and Table 1, **Notes 5** and **6**) [7].

4 Notes

1. Trypsin solution should only be used when it is freshly made from frozen powder due to suspected autodigestion after being dissolved in AB buffer. The suppliers also provide vials with 20 μg if few colonies are characterized by MS.

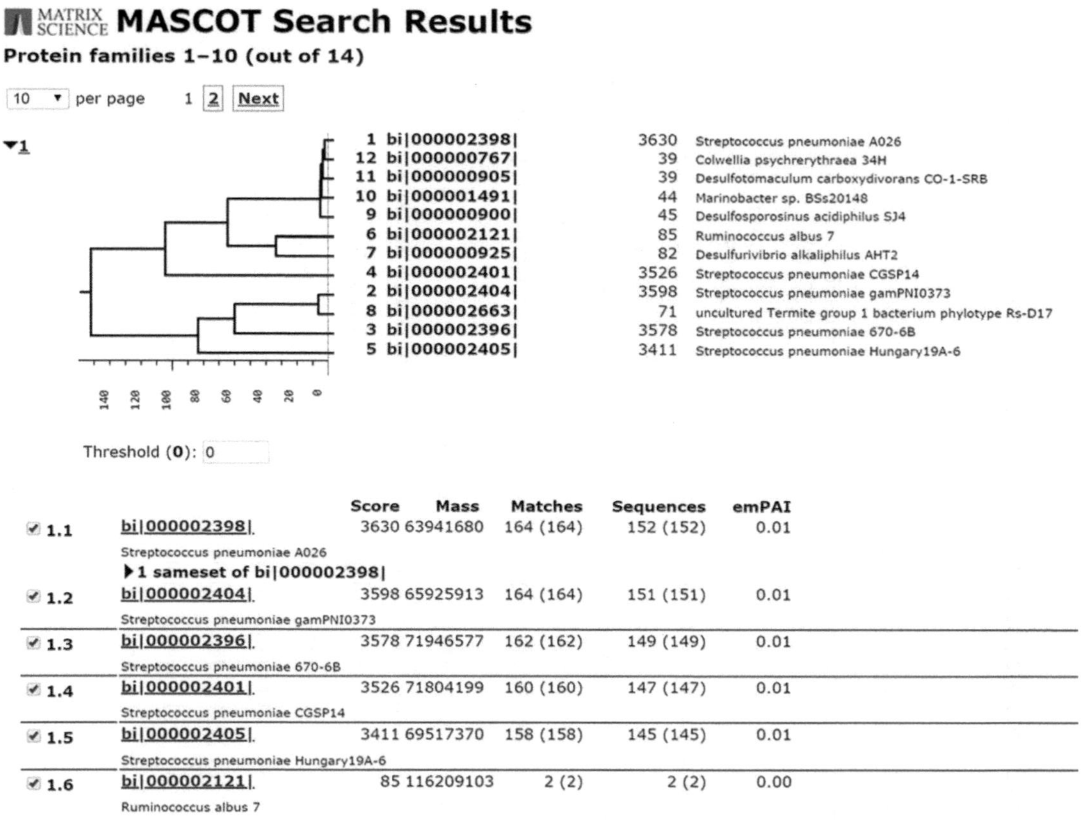

Fig. 1 Representative result of Mascot database search for bacterial identification from single colony of *Streptococcus pneumoniae.* "Score" represents the Mascot score of combined peptides identified; "Mass" signifies the whole proteome mass in Daltons; "Matches" signifies the number of peptides identified (redundant); "Sequences" equals the number of peptide sequences identified (nonredundant); "emPAI" is calculated as [ten to the power of (the number of observed peptides divided by the number of observable peptides) minus one] [5, 6]

2. Digestion can be extended overnight without influencing the result. However, in this case, overdigestion should be avoided by adding 1% FA (for final FA concentration of 0.1%) the following morning.
3. The final digests must be filtered to prevent materials (such as agar pieces for *Streptococcus pneumoniae* colony) that might clog the nano-LC system.
4. In LC-MS/MS, attention should be paid to sample carryover [2, 4]; therefore, performing a column wash between samples is suggested.
5. The database to be used should be specially produced and annotated for bacterial identification using the whole proteome of individual bacteria [7] (*see* Table 1).
6. If carryover is suspected, performing additional and harsher washes may be necessary [5].

Table 1
Representative results for bacterial identification of single colonies by liquid chromatography–tandem mass spectrometry (LC-MS/MS) using reference strains[a]

<table>
<tr><th>Reference strain/test</th><th>Sample load</th><th>Code</th><th>Score</th><th>Mass</th><th>Matches</th><th>Sequences</th><th>emPAI</th><th>ID</th></tr>
<tr><td>Sal En-01</td><td>1/10</td><td>bi|000002146|</td><td>117752</td><td>147660248</td><td>5211 (5211)</td><td>3450 (3450)</td><td>0.09</td><td>Salmonella enterica subsp. enterica serovar Enteritidis str. P125109</td></tr>
<tr><td>Sal En-02</td><td>1/10</td><td>bi|000002146|</td><td>111068</td><td>147660248</td><td>4877 (4877)</td><td>3322 (3322)</td><td>0.09</td><td>Salmonella enterica subsp. enterica serovar Enteritidis str. P125109</td></tr>
<tr><td>Sal En-03</td><td>1/10</td><td>bi|000002146|</td><td>116227</td><td>147660248</td><td>5040 (5040)</td><td>3473 (3473)</td><td>0.09</td><td>Salmonella enterica subsp. enterica serovar Enteritidis str. P125109</td></tr>
<tr><td>E coli-01</td><td>1/10</td><td>bi|000001032|</td><td>74586</td><td>174582699</td><td>3231 (3231)</td><td>1606 (1606)</td><td>0.04</td><td>Escherichia coli O157:H7 str. Sakai [EHEC]</td></tr>
<tr><td>E coli-02</td><td>1/10</td><td>bi|000001032|</td><td>41658</td><td>174582699</td><td>2075 (2075)</td><td>980 (980)</td><td>0.02</td><td>Escherichia coli O157:H7 str. Sakai [EHEC]</td></tr>
<tr><td>E coli-03</td><td>1/10</td><td>bi|000001033|</td><td>38066</td><td>174445670</td><td>1858 (1858)</td><td>945 (945)</td><td>0.02</td><td>Escherichia coli O157:H7 str. TW14359 [EHEC]</td></tr>
<tr><td>NM-01</td><td>1/10</td><td>bi|000001756|</td><td>27472</td><td>64421788</td><td>1008 (1008)</td><td>918 (918)</td><td>0.06</td><td>Neisseria meningitidis H44/76</td></tr>
<tr><td>NM-02</td><td>1/10</td><td>bi|000001756|</td><td>32837</td><td>64421788</td><td>1168 (1168)</td><td>1061 (1061)</td><td>0.07</td><td>Neisseria meningitidis H44/76</td></tr>
<tr><td>NM-03</td><td>1/10</td><td>bi|000001751|</td><td>16476</td><td>63825740</td><td>614 (614)</td><td>552 (552)</td><td>0.04</td><td>Neisseria meningitidis 8013</td></tr>
<tr><td>SA-01</td><td>1/10</td><td>bi|000002279|</td><td>7764</td><td>88864960</td><td>339 (339)</td><td>323 (323)</td><td>0.02</td><td>Staphylococcus aureus 04-02981</td></tr>
<tr><td>SA-02</td><td>1/10</td><td>bi|000002279|</td><td>28094</td><td>88864960</td><td>1018 (1018)</td><td>933 (933)</td><td>0.04</td><td>Staphylococcus aureus 04-02981</td></tr>
<tr><td>SA-03</td><td>1/10</td><td>bi|000002303|</td><td>28546</td><td>90734925</td><td>1030 (1030)</td><td>943 (943)</td><td>0.04</td><td>Staphylococcus aureus subsp. aureus Mu3</td></tr>
<tr><td>49619-01</td><td>1/20</td><td>bi|000002408|</td><td>5264</td><td>66843273</td><td>162 (162)</td><td>141 (141)</td><td>0.01</td><td>Streptococcus pneumoniae JJA</td></tr>
<tr><td>49619-02</td><td>1/20</td><td>bi|000002397|</td><td>1982</td><td>69034182</td><td>77 (77)</td><td>73 (73)</td><td>0</td><td>Streptococcus pneumoniae 70,585</td></tr>
</table>

49619-03	1/20	bi|000002407|	1465	64899212	50 (50)	44 (44)	0	*Streptococcus pneumoniae* INV200
6318-01	1/20	bi|000002411|	385	63295868	11 (11)	9 (9)	0	*Streptococcus pneumoniae* R6
6318-02	1/20	bi|000002412|	634	60575524	16 (16)	16 (16)	0	*Streptococcus pneumoniae* SPN034156
6318-03	1/20	bi|000002411|	233	63295868	5 (5)	5 (5)	0	*Streptococcus pneumoniae* R6
49619-01	1/10	bi|000002398|	3669	63941680	158 (158)	137 (137)	0.01	*Streptococcus pneumoniae* A026
49619-02	1/10	bi|000002398|	2500	63941680	115 (115)	98 (98)	0.01	*Streptococcus pneumoniae* A026
49619-03	1/10	bi|000002396|	1903	71946577	74 (74)	62 (62)	0	*Streptococcus pneumoniae* 670-6B
6318-02	1/10	bi|000002399|	1064	68963964	57 (57)	51 (51)	0	*Streptococcus pneumoniae* AP200
6318-02	1/10	bi|000002399|	1064	68963964	57 (57)	51 (51)	0	*Streptococcus pneumoniae* AP200
6318-03	1/10	bi|000002409|	441	61461726	19 (19)	19 (19)	0	*Streptococcus pneumoniae* OXC141
49619-A	1/10	bi|000002396|	1501	71946577	87 (87)	84 (84)	0	*Streptococcus pneumoniae* 670-6B
49619-B	1/10	bi|000002419|	1629	68486833	82 (82)	79 (79)	0	*Streptococcus pneumoniae* TCH8431/19A
49619-C	1/10	bi|000002415|	1098	61183704	49 (49)	47 (47)	0	*Streptococcus pneumoniae* SPN994039
49619-D	1/10	bi|000002406|	1079	63895733	59 (59)	58 (58)	0	*Streptococcus pneumoniae* INV104
6318-A	1/10	bi|000002398|	5348	63941680	243 (243)	227 (227)	0.01	*Streptococcus pneumoniae* A026
6318-B	1/10	bi|000002420|	2311	67432288	98 (98)	92 (92)	0.01	*Streptococcus pneumoniae* TIGR4
6318-C	1/10	bi|000002398|	3630	63941680	164 (164)	152 (152)	0.01	*Streptococcus pneumoniae* A026
6318-D	1/10	bi|000002420|	2642	67432288	103 (103)	99 (99)	0.01	*Streptococcus pneumoniae* TIGR4
49619-X	1/10	bi|000002396|	5193	71946577	213 (213)	188 (188)	0.01	*Streptococcus pneumoniae* 670-6B
49619-Y	1/10	bi|000002398|	5203	63941680	215 (215)	194 (194)	0.01	*Streptococcus pneumoniae* A026

(continued)

Table 1
(continued)

<table>
<tr><th>Reference strain/test</th><th>Sample load</th><th>Code</th><th>Score</th><th>Mass</th><th>Matches</th><th>Sequences</th><th>emPAI</th><th>ID</th></tr>
<tr><td>49619-Z</td><td>1/10</td><td>bi|000002396|</td><td>3019</td><td>71946577</td><td>122 (122)</td><td>109 (109)</td><td>0.01</td><td>Streptococcus pneumoniae 670-6B</td></tr>
<tr><td>6318-X</td><td>1/10</td><td>bi|000002418|</td><td>756</td><td>65496826</td><td>40 (40)</td><td>38 (38)</td><td>0</td><td>Streptococcus pneumoniae Taiwan19F-14</td></tr>
<tr><td>6318-Y</td><td>1/10</td><td>bi|000002419|</td><td>1127</td><td>68486833</td><td>53 (53)</td><td>51 (51)</td><td>0</td><td>Streptococcus pneumoniae TCH8431/19A</td></tr>
<tr><td>6318-Z</td><td>1/10</td><td>bi|000002403|</td><td>1486</td><td>66890036</td><td>64 (64)</td><td>61 (61)</td><td>0</td><td>Streptococcus pneumoniae G54</td></tr>
</table>

[a]Sal En, ***Salmonella enterica*** subsp. ***enterica serovar Enteritidis***; E coli, ***Escherichia coli***; NM, ***Neisseria meningitidis***; SA, ***Staphylococcus aureus***; 49619 and 6138 are two ATCC ***Streptococcus pneumoniae*** reference strains. Tests were repeated at different points during cell culture with different amount of sample loaded onto the nano-LC-MS/MS system (represented by 1, 2, 3, 4; A, B, C, D; or X, Y, Z). "Code" is an assigned code for the individual bacterial strain used; "Score" represents the Mascot score of combined peptides identified; "Mass" signifies the whole proteome mass in Daltons; "Matches" signifies the number of peptides identified (redundant); "Sequences" equals the number of peptide sequences identified (nonredundant); "emPAI" is calculated as [ten to the power of (the number of observed peptides divided by the number of observable peptides) minus one] [5]; "ID" denotes the strain name used in database creation. Some emPAI values were shown as "0" due to the limit of the significant number of digits employed by Mascot

Acknowledgments

We thank Stuart McCorrister and Chris Grant in the Proteomics Core, National Microbiology Laboratory, Public Health Agency of Canada for creating the database and running the MS.

References

1. Cheng K, Chui H, Domish L et al (2016) Recent development of mass spectrometry and proteomics applications in identification and typing of bacteria. Proteomics Clin Appl 10:346–357. https://doi.org/10.1002/prca.201500086
2. Cheng K, Sloan A, Peterson L, McCorrister S et al (2014) Comparative study of traditional flagellum serotyping and liquid chromatography-tandem mass spectrometry-based flagellum typing with clinical *Escherichia coli* isolates. J Clin Microbiol 52(6):2275–2278. https://doi.org/10.1128/JCM.00174-14
3. Chui H, Chan M, Hernandez D et al (2015) Rapid, sensitive, and specific *Escherichia coli* H antigen typing by matrix-assisted laser desorption ionization-time of flight-based peptide mass fingerprinting. J Clin Microbiol 53(8):2480–2485. https://doi.org/10.1128/JCM.00593-15
4. Cheng K, She YM, Chui H et al (2016) Mass spectrometry-based *Escherichia coli* H antigen/flagella typing: validation and comparison with traditional serotyping. Clin Chem 62(6):839–847. https://doi.org/10.1373/clinchem.2015.244236
5. Cheng K, Sloan A, McCorrister S et al (2014) Quality evaluation of LC-MS/MS-based *E. coli* H antigen typing (MS-H) through label-free quantitative data analysis in a clinical sample setup. Proteomics Clin Appl 8:963–970. https://doi.org/10.1002/prca.201400019
6. Ishihama Y, Oda Y, Tabata T et al (2005) Exponentially modified protein abundance index (emPAI) for estimationof absolute protein amount in proteomics by the number of sequencedpeptides per protein. Mol Cell Proteomics 4(9):1265–1272. https://doi.org/10.1074/mcp.M500061-MCP200
7. Tracz DM, McCorrister SJ, Chong PM et al (2013) A simple shotgun proteomics method for rapid bacterial identification. J Microbiol Methods 94(1):54–57. https://doi.org/10.1016/j.mimet.2013.04.008

Chapter 11

Bead-Based Flow-Cytometric Cell Counting of Live and Dead Bacteria

Fang Ou, Cushla McGoverin, Joni White, Simon Swift, and Frédérique Vanholsbeeck

Abstract

Flow cytometry (FCM) is based on the detection of scattered light and fluorescence to identify cells with characteristics of interest. Many flow cytometers cannot precisely control the flow through its interrogation point and hence the volume and concentration of the sample cannot be immediately obtained. Here we describe the optimization and evaluation of a bead-based method for absolute cell counting applicable to basic flow cytometers without specialized counting features. Prior to the application of this method to an unknown concentration of a species of bacteria, a calibration experiment should be completed to characterize limits of detection and range of linearity with respect to the plate count method. To demonstrate the calibration process, mixtures of *Escherichia coli* or *Staphylococcus aureus* with proportions of live and dead cells ranging from 0% to 100% were prepared. These samples were stained using nucleic acid-binding dyes, and 6 μm reference beads were added (LIVE/DEAD® BacLight kit). The calibration samples were analyzed using bead-based FCM as well as the agar plate count method, and the results from both methods were compared.

Key words Bacteria, Bacterial cell enumeration, Flow cytometry, Counting beads, Fluorescence, Detection

1 Introduction

Enumeration of both live and dead bacteria is desirable in many fields of microbiological research and for the monitoring of food safety and public health. One highly ranked assessment of bacterial viability is membrane integrity [1], and for this purpose the nucleic acid-binding dyes SYTO 9 and PI are commonly used as they differentially stain live and dead bacteria, respectively [2–6]. The distinct fluorescence emission wavelengths of SYTO 9 and PI may be detected using flow cytometry (FCM) to identify live and dead bacterial cells. The key advantage of FCM over traditional agar plate count and fluorescence microscopy methods is the capacity

Federico Iovino (ed.), *Streptococcus pneumoniae: Methods and Protocols*, Methods in Molecular Biology, vol. 1968, https://doi.org/10.1007/978-1-4939-9199-0_11,

to acquire single-cell information in large sample sets with comparatively little effort.

Although FCM can measure the relative proportion of cell populations in a mixture, not all flow cytometers are able to acquire the concentration of the cells. This is because many flow cytometers are unable to precisely control or monitor the sample flow through the interrogation point [7]. Hence, the number of particles analyzed in one measurement cannot be directly correlated with a specific sample volume from which to calculate the concentration. The simplest, most reliable and low-cost way of obtaining absolute concentration of cells in these instances is to use reference beads [7]. The bead-based FCM method has been applied in previous studies where the counts of live bacteria were compared with the results obtained from agar plate counts [4, 8] and hemocytometer counts [9]. However, these studies did not investigate a wide range of bacterial concentrations or different ratios of live and dead cells. Furthermore, the counts of dead bacterial cells were not evaluated.

The bead-based FCM counting method for enumerating live and dead bacteria has been described by the manufacturer since the release of the SYTO 9 and PI staining kit more than one decade ago [6]. However, the methods outlined did not include numerous precautions that should be taken or the associated experimental error. We have addressed these issues by evaluating the bead-based FCM method in conjunction with the use of SYTO 9 and PI, to quantify varying ratios of live and dead *Escherichia coli* (ATCC 25922) [10] and *Staphylococcus aureus* (ATCC 6538). In this chapter, we outline the steps required to calibrate the bead-based FCM method for the gram-negative rod (ca. 0.5 by 2 μm) *E. coli*, as well as the processing steps for samples with unknown concentration. The calibration experiment determines the limit of detection of the bead-based FCM method for a combination of the flow cytometer machine, settings, and bacterial species; and allows for inspection of the linearity between the bead-based FCM and plate count results. For concentrations within the linear range, it is not necessary to obtain a standard curve to calibrate FCM counts to plate counts. For *E. coli*, it is possible to count live and dead cells over a wide concentration range, from 10^4 to 10^8 bacteria/mL [10]. Bacteria with different physiology [e.g., gram-positive cocci like *S. aureus* (ca. 0.6 μm diameter)] can be studied but with minor protocol changes such as culture conditions and location of the FCM gates. Before the application of this method to new bacterial sample types, initial calibration experiments should be performed using the species to be tested. This bead-based FCM method is highly adaptable and has the potential to be extended to a wider concentration range and to study other bacterial species and strains, e.g., *Streptococcus pneumoniae* and methicillin-resistant *Staphylococcus aureus* (MRSA).

2 Materials

Sterilized saline solution (0.85% w/v) is used in sample preparation and washing. All buffers and media are autoclave-sterilized and the aseptic technique is followed.

2.1 Bacterial Sample Preparation

1. *Escherichia coli* strain ATCC 25922 (American Type Culture Collection, Virginia, USA) (*see* **Note 1**). For long-term storage of bacteria, a 1:1 mixture of overnight bacterial broth culture with sterile 50% (v/v) glycerol is made and stored in cryovials at −80 °C. The bacterial stock of *E. coli* (ATCC 25922) is therefore stored at −80 °C in 25% glycerol.
2. Difco tryptic soy broth (TSB): 30 g/L of a premixed TSB powder that produces a broth containing 17 g/L of casein (pancreatic digest), 3 g/L of soya peptone (papaic digest), 5 g/L of sodium chloride, 2.5 g/L of dipotassium phosphate, and 2.5 g/L of dextrose.
3. Difco tryptic soy agar (TSA) plates (*see* **Note 2**): 30 g/L of premixed TSB powder and 15 g/L of Difco agar.
4. 50 mL V-bottom centrifuge tubes (*see* **Note 3**).
5. 70% v/v isopropyl alcohol, diluted from 100% with sterile saline.
6. Saline (0.85% w/v): 8.5 g/L of sodium chloride.

2.2 Fluorescent Dye Staining and Microsphere Protocol

1. BacLight LIVE/DEAD Bacterial Viability and Counting kit (Invitrogen, Molecular Probes, Carlsbad, CA, USA; L34856). The kit contains a microsphere suspension (1×10^8 beads/mL, 6 μm bead diameter) and two nucleic acid dyes 3.34 mM SYTO 9 and 20 mM propidium iodide (PI) that label live and dead bacteria, respectively. The manufacturer recommends that the stock solutions are refrigerated (2–6 °C) [6].
2. Working solution of 0.0334 mM SYTO 9 to stain the bacterial samples: for eight samples, add 4.5 μL of 3.34 mM SYTO 9 to 445.5 μL of saline (*see* **Note 4**).
3. Working solution of 0.4 mM PI to stain the bacterial samples: for eight samples, add 9 μL of 20 mM PI to 441 μL of saline (*see* **Note 4**).
4. Amber or similar microcentrifuge tubes (*see* **Note 5**).

2.3 Flow Cytometry Equipment and Materials

1. Flow Cytometer (LSR II Flow Cytometer, BD Biosciences, San Jose, CA, USA) with 488 nm excitation laser (20 mW power is used in this method).
2. Flow cytometer analysis software (BD FACSDIVA software package, BD Biosciences, San Jose, CA, USA) (*see* **Note 6**).
3. 5 mL polystyrene round-bottom tubes for FCM analysis.

3 Methods

Homogenous bacterial suspensions are produced via ca. 5 s of vortexing in all instances prior to pipetting, unless otherwise stated.

3.1 Bacterial Culture

1. To recover bacteria from frozen storage, ice from the stock tube is removed with a sterile plastic loop and streaked onto a culture plate (TSA) to obtain single colonies after incubation. For *E. coli,* growth is overnight at 37 °C.
2. Transfer the growth from a single colony to 10 mL of sterile TSB inside a 50 mL V-bottom centrifuge tube and incubate overnight at 37 °C with orbital shaking (200 rpm).
3. Following overnight incubation, confirm that the culture has reached more than ca. 2×10^9 CFU/mL; for *E. coli* this has an optical density (OD) of at least 1.8 at 600 nm (path length 1 cm).
4. Prepare a subculture of exponentially growing cells by adding 0.5 mL of the overnight culture into 9.5 mL of fresh TSB inside a 50 mL V-bottom centrifuge tube and continue the incubation for approximately 1 h. End the incubation when the subculture grows to reach ca. 4×10^8 CFU/mL, for *E. coli* this has an OD between 0.5 and 0.6 at 600 nm (path length 1 cm).
5. Harvest cells from the subculture by centrifugation (4302 × *g*, 10 min, 21 °C) followed by removal of supernatant (*see* **Note 7**), and resuspension in 3 mL of saline to ca. 10^9 CFU/mL.

3.2 Preparation of Calibration Samples

1. Dilute 1 mL of the harvested subculture with 9 mL of saline to produce the live bacterial suspension. This gives a concentration of ca. 10^8 CFU/mL. Then dilute another 1 mL of the harvested subculture with 9 mL of 70% isopropyl alcohol to produce the dead bacterial suspension.
2. Incubate the live and dead bacterial suspensions for 15 min at room temperature (20 °C) with orbital shaking at 200 rpm (*see* **Note 8**).
3. During incubation (Subheading 3.2, **step 2**), dilute 100 μL of the harvested subculture (from Subheading 3.1, **step 6**) by 10^6 times in saline to ensure countable colonies. Plate 100 μL aliquots onto triplicate TSA plates (three technical replicates) and label these plates as "A." Then dilute 100 μL of the live bacterial suspension (from Subheading 3.2, **step 1**) by 10^5 times in saline. Plate 100 μL aliquots onto triplicate TSA plates and label these plates as "B."
4. After incubation (from Subheading 3.2, **step 2**), dilute 100 μL of the live bacterial suspension by 10^5 times in saline. Plate 100 μL onto triplicate TSA plates. Label these plates as "C" (*see* **Note 9**).

5. Harvest the live and dead cells via three cycles of the washing process: centrifugation (4302 × *g*, 10 min, 21 °C) followed by removal of the supernatant and resuspension in 20 mL of saline.
6. After the final wash, resuspend the live and dead cells separately in 10 mL of saline. Dilute 100 μL of the live bacterial suspension by 10^5 times in saline. Plate 100 μL onto triplicate TSA plates and label these plates as "D" (*see* **Note 10**).
7. Plate 100 μL of the undiluted dead bacterial suspension onto duplicate TSA plates (two technical replicates) to confirm all cells are dead. Label these plates as "dead."
8. To obtain the live and dead bacterial stock solutions each with a concentration of ca. 1×10^8 bacteria/mL, further dilute the live and dead bacterial solutions until the appropriate optical density is reached (for *E. coli* it is ca. 0.2 at 600 nm).
9. Make calibration samples by using the live and dead bacterial stock solutions and mixing them in various live–dead ratios. For example, eight samples can be mixed that contain 0%, 2.5%, 5%, 10%, 25%, 50%, 75%, and 100% live bacteria. To make 3 mL of the 2.5% live bacterial sample, it will contain 75 μL of the live bacterial stock solution and 2925 μL of the dead bacterial stock solution.

3.3 Preparation of Samples with Unknown Concentration

After the characterization of the limit of detection of the FCM method, environmental samples or samples produced by others can be analyzed.

1. To analyze bacterial samples with unknown live–dead concentration, suspend the cells in a nonfluorescent solution free of particulate matter (saline was used in this method) to minimize noise in FCM measurements.

3.4 Fluorescent Dye Staining and Microsphere Protocol

1. The live and dead bacterial samples can be stored in an icebox for no more than 1.5 h prior to the fluorescent dye staining step.
2. Allow time for the stock dye and reference bead solutions to warm to room temperature before use. Visually check that the dyes have fully melted.
3. Centrifuge the tubes of SYTO 9 and PI for 1 min at 7826 × *g* (*see* **Note 11**).
4. Make working solutions of 0.0334 mM SYTO 9 and 0.4 mM PI, prepared by the dilution of stock dyes in saline.
5. For staining each sample, aliquot 50 μL of the working solution of SYTO 9 and 50 μL of the working solution of PI into an empty microcentrifuge tube.

6. Before dispensing beads from the bottle, sonicate the microsphere suspension for 10 min in a water bath sonicator followed by a series of gentle inversions of the tube or low speed vortexing at *c.* 500 rpm (*see* **Note 12**). Visually inspect that the suspension is homogenous and ensure there is no clumping of beads at the bottom of the bottle.
7. Add 10 μL of the microsphere suspension to each amber tube containing SYTO 9 and PI.
8. Remove the bacterial mixtures from the icebox and aliquot 900 μL of each mixture into an amber microcentrifuge tube containing the dyes and beads.
9. Vortex the stained samples gently at 500 rpm for 15 min prior to measurement on the flow cytometer.

3.5 Flow Cytometry

The calibration samples need to be plated, and this should be done in parallel to their measurement on the flow cytometer (*see* **Note 13**).

1. Choose the laser source that matches the excitation range of the fluorescent dyes used. In this method a 488 nm laser with 20 mW power was used as it excites both SYTO 9 and PI.
2. Choose specific fluorescence cutoff and bandpass filters that match the emission range of the dyes used and try to minimize spectral overlap of the collection channels. In this method, SYTO 9 fluorescence was collected using a 505 nm longpass filter and a bandpass filter with 530/30 nm transmission. The PI fluorescence was collected using a 685 nm longpass filter and a bandpass filter with 695/40 nm transmission.
3. Configure the flow cytometer settings for data collection: Establish a threshold for the flow cytometer based on the analysis of a blank sample, in this method saline was used as the blank sample and the threshold was set to side scatter (SSC) at 200. To display the entire data collected, adjust the photomultiplier tube voltage so that both the bacterial populations and beads were on scale in a SSC vs forward scatter (FSC) plot. To further minimize noise, only SYTO 9-positive events were included in the bacterial analysis as live and dead bacteria are both stained by SYTO 9. The number of SYTO 9-positive events can be plotted as a function of their PI intensity, from which live and dead cells can be initially identified (Fig. 1). Perform the gating for analysis of live and dead bacterial populations in the red fluorescence vs green fluorescence dot plot, an example is shown in Fig. 2. To monitor the consistency of the bead count as a function of time, incorporate a time histogram as shown in Fig. 3.
4. Aliquot 300 μL of each stained bacterial sample into three FCM tubes (three technical replicates).

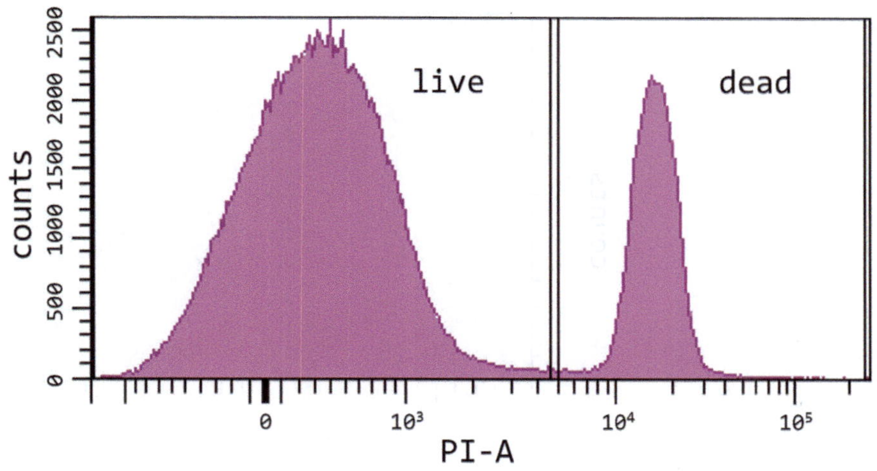

Fig. 1 Distinction between live and dead bacterial populations. Histogram shows the frequency of SYTO 9-positive events as a function of the intensity of their PI signal. This plot is useful for the visual inspection of live and dead cell populations, which display low and high PI intensities ("PI-A"), respectively

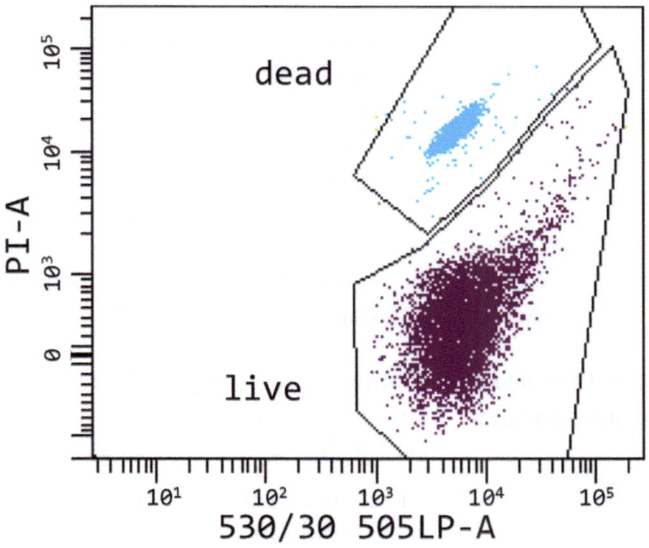

Fig. 2 Flow cytometry analysis of a sample containing both live and dead bacteria. Gating is performed in a flow cytometry cytogram of the PI ("PI-A") versus SYTO 9 ("530/30505LP-A") fluorescence. The top box gates the dead bacterial cells whereas the bottom box gates the live bacterial cells as well as those that are injured which show staining by both SYTO 9 and PI

5. Homogenize the sample by gently vortexing the sample at ca. 500 rpm prior to measuring.
6. Measure each sample using a flow rate of ca. 6 μL/min for a duration of 150 s (*see* **Note 14**).

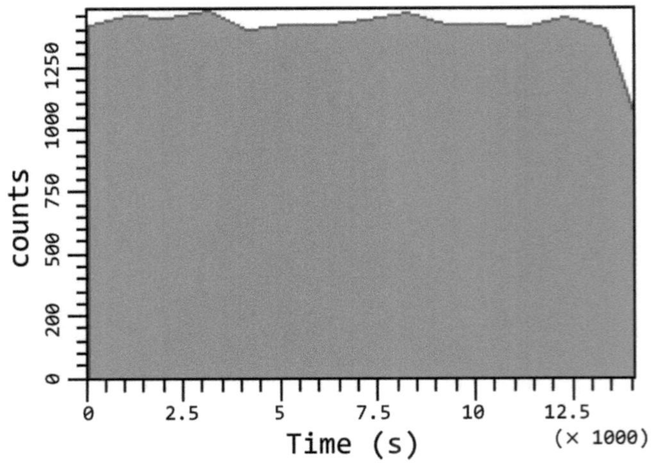

Fig. 3 The flow rate of reference beads during sample acquisition. Histogram shows the variation in bead counts over a sample acquisition period of 150 s. This plot is useful for monitoring the flow rate of reference beads, which gives an indication of sample flow rate during measurement

7. Calculate the absolute concentration of bacterial populations (*see* **Note 15**) and find the mean and standard error for each sample.
8. Data processing and analysis: calculations for the FCM and plate count data can be processed using Microsoft Excel or a comparable spreadsheet software. Regression plots and statistics such as R^2 have been calculated via Python programming using the numpy and matplotlib packages. Other programs may also be used, such as R, Matlab, and Excel.

3.6 Agar Plate Count of Calibration Samples

Plating is only required for the calibration samples, and these should be plated unstained and in parallel to their measurements on the flow cytometer (*see* **Note 13**).

1. Dilute 100 μL of the unstained bacterial mixtures and plate 100 μL onto triplicate TSA plates (three technical replicates for each calibration sample) (*see* **Note 16**).
2. Incubate all plates for a length of time and temperature suitable for the bacterial species. For example, in this method, the *E. coli* plates are incubated overnight at 37 °C.
3. Enumerate the colonies grown on each plate and calculate the mean bacteria/mL and the standard error for each sample.
4. Compare the FCM and plate count results for the concentration of live and dead (*see* **Note 17**) bacteria.

4 Notes

1. *Escherichia coli* is used as it is a widely adopted test organism in microbiology and is also the most rigorously studied species of bacteria [11]. The bead-based FCM method has also been successfully applied to *Staphylococcus aureus*. Other species (e.g., *Streptococcus pneumoniae*) may also be used with minor changes (such as the culture conditions, optical density reading requirements and FCM gating). Prior to applying the method to a different bacterial species, it is recommended to first characterize the relationship between optical density and the CFU/mL of bacteria.
2. To reduce condensation, it is recommended to take the TSA plates out of the fridge one night before the experiment to allow time for the plates to reach room temperature. If the plates are used cold, condensation will form and the plates will be wet; this could lead to the merging of colonies and difficulties with colony counting. Alternatively, the plates can be warmed in an incubator or within the updraft field of a Bunsen flame prior to use, which also helps reduce condensation. In all cases, continue to spread the bacterial solution evenly until the plate is dry.
3. A maximum volume of 10 mL in the 50 mL tube is maintained to allow for constant and adequate aeration.
4. Making a working solution of the SYTO 9 and PI dyes improves the accuracy of pipetting as it avoids the need to pipet small volumes such as 0.5 μL. Note that the volumes specified for staining $N = 8$ samples is enough to stain nine samples (450 μL total of each working solution of dye; 50 μL of each stock dye is required for each sample). Making enough stock dye for $N + 1$ samples minimizes the pipetting of inaccurate dye volumes, especially if droplets of dye are stuck to walls of the tube or pipette tip.
5. The stained samples will be fluorescent; hence, precautions should be taken to ensure light exposure is minimal until analyses are conducted. The use of amber tubes is preferred, these shield from ambient light and reduce photobleaching of the dyes.
6. Other software such as FlowJo (FlowJo LLC, Ashland Oregon, USA) and the Flowing Software (Cell Imaging Core of the Turku Centre for Biotechnology, Turku, Finland) can also be used to analyze the .fcs files acquired by flow cytometry.
7. To avoid losing bacterial cells along with the supernatant, all supernatant removal steps should be performed immediately after centrifugation ends. The supernatant is removed by

carefully decanting off the liquid immediately following centrifugation, while the bacterial cells are tightly packed into a pellet.

8. Complete killing of *E. coli* is achievable in 15 min of incubation, the time required for other species of bacteria may be different.
9. By comparing the plate count results from "C" plates with that of "A" and "B" plates, the percentage change in bacterial concentration caused by the 15 min-long incubation can be estimated.
10. By comparing the plate count results from "D" plates with that of "C" plates, the percentage change in bacterial concentration caused by washing the samples three times can be estimated.
11. Centrifuging the bottles of SYTO 9 and PI ensures that there are no droplets stuck onto the side walls and thus makes it easier to pipet from and minimizes the waste of dyes.
12. Be careful to avoid strong vortexing and shaking which induces foam formation [12, 13]. The micro-air bubbles formed will attract the beads, and subsequently skew the volume and concentration of the beads pipetted into the sample [12, 13]. If foaming occurs, rest the bottle to allow time for the foam to disappear and continue the experiment using a different bottle of beads. Using different bottles of beads is not a significant source of variation for these experiments [10].
13. It is recommended to perform plating and FCM measurements of the calibration samples in parallel, to minimize differences in bacterial concentration due to growth that occurs between different measurement times.
14. In FCM, coincidence refers to the aggregation of two or more cells as they pass through the detection point, thus resulting in slight underestimation of cell counts. Measuring on a low flow rate minimizes the occurrence of coincidence, and measuring for 150 s ensures that a substantial number of events are captured in the analysis.

    If the aim is to detect low levels of bacteria at concentrations of ca. 10^4 bacteria/mL or lower, then the technique can be modified to improve the sensitivity of the method. For example, to ensure that enough events are captured despite the decreased concentration of particles, the flow rate of the flow cytometer and duration of measurement can be increased. Furthermore, the volume of beads added can be decreased to avoid saturating the system with bead signals.
15. The concentration of the live or dead bacterial population can be calculated using the formula below [6, 10, 14]:

$$\text{Conc. of bacterial population} = \frac{\text{\#events in population region}}{\text{\#events in bead region}} \times \text{conc.of beads} \times \text{dilution factor}$$

where the "conc. of beads" refers to the bead concentration in the entire sample volume and the "dilution factor" refers to the dilution of the bacterial sample. For calculating the concentration of live bacteria, "# events in population region" refers to the cells stained by SYTO 9 but not PI as determined by the FCM procedure. To calculate the concentration of dead bacteria, "# events in population region" refers to the PI-stained cells.

16. Dilute the bacterial samples such that about 30–300 colonies are expected on the final plates. As the final samples are made by mixing live and dead stock bacterial solutions with a concentration of ca. 1×10^8 bacteria/mL, the bacterial mixtures containing more than 30% of live bacteria should therefore be diluted 10^5 times with 100 μL plated. The bacterial mixtures containing less than 30% of live bacteria should only be diluted 10^4 times, as these contain more dead bacterial cells which do not grow.

17. Although dead bacteria do not grow and hence do not form colonies, the concentration of dead bacteria can nonetheless be indirectly estimated from plate counts. This is required in the calibration of the bead-based FCM method to characterize its limit of detection and range of linearity with respect to the plate count method. To achieve this, the harvested subculture and the ten times diluted subculture were plated and labeled as "A" and "B," respectively. The average counts obtained from plates "A" and "B" can then be used to determine the concentration of bacteria killed by incubation in 70% isopropyl alcohol. Subsequently, by considering the dilution factors used and the percentage uncertainties introduced by the 15 min-long incubation step and the washing cycles that followed, the "concentration of dead bacteria" in the dead bacterial stock solution (ca. 10^8 bacteria/mL according to optical density measurements) can be calculated. Then, knowing the volume of dead bacterial stock solution added ("vol. of dead bacteria added") to each calibration sample, the final "expected concentration of dead bacteria" can be calculated using the formula below:

$$\text{Expected conc.of dead bacteria} = \frac{\text{conc.of dead bacteria} \times \text{vol.of dead bacteria added}}{\text{vol.of mixture}}$$

Acknowledgments

We are grateful to the New Zealand Ministry of Business, Innovation and Employment for funding the Food Safe; real time bacterial count (UOAX1411) research programme. This work is in partial fulfilment of Fang Ou's PhD thesis, who is grateful for the University of Auckland Doctoral Scholarship, the Todd Foundation Award for Excellence, the RHT Bates Scholarship and the Claude McCarthy Fellowship. Joni White is grateful for the Maurice and Phyllis Paykel Trust Research Scholarship in Health Sciences and the New Zealand Meat Industry Postgraduate Scholarship. The authors thank Stephen Edgar, Dr. Julia Robertson, Zak Whiting, and Janesha Perera for their laboratory support.

References

1. Vives-Rego J, Lebaron P, Nebe-von Caron G (2000) Current and future applications of flow cytometry in aquatic microbiology. FEMS Microbiol Rev 24(4):429–448
2. Berney M, Hammes F, Bosshard F, Weilenmann H-U, Egli T (2007) Assessment and interpretation of bacterial viability by using the LIVE/DEAD BacLight Kit in combination with flow cytometry. Appl Environ Microbiol 73(10):3283–3290
3. Duedu KO, French CE (2017) Two-colour fluorescence fluorimetric analysis for direct quantification of bacteria and its application in monitoring bacterial growth in cellulose degradation systems. J Microbiol Methods 135:85–92
4. He S, Hong X, Huang T, Zhang W, Zhou Y, Wu L, Yan X (2017) Rapid quantification of live/dead lactic acid bacteria in probiotic products using high-sensitivity flow cytometry. Methods Appl Fluoresc 5(2):024002
5. Stocks SM (2004) Mechanism and use of the commercially available viability stain BacLight. Cytometry A 61(2):189–195
6. ThermoFisher Scientific (2004) LIVE/DEAD ® BacLight™ bacterial viability and counting kit (L34856) Product Information. https://tools.thermofisher.com/content/sfs/manuals/mp34856.pdf. Accessed 22 Feb 2018
7. Gasol JM, Del Giorgio PA (2000) Using flow cytometry for counting natural planktonic bacteria and understanding the structure of planktonic bacterial communities. Sci Mar 64 (2):197–224
8. Alsharif R, Godfrey W (2002) Bacterial detection and live/dead discrimination by flow cytometry. BD Biosciences. https://www.bdbiosciences.com/documents/Bacterial_Detection_Live_Dead.pdf. Accessed 3 Mar 2018
9. Peniuk GT, Schnurr PJ, Allen DG (2016) Identification and quantification of suspended algae and bacteria populations using flow cytometry: applications for algae biofuel and biochemical growth systems. J Appl Phycol 28 (1):95–104
10. Ou F, McGoverin C, Swift S, Vanholsbeeck F (2017) Absolute bacterial cell enumeration using flow cytometry. J Appl Microbiol 123 (2):464–477
11. Cooper GM (ed) (2000) The cell, 2nd edn. Sinauer Associates, Sunderland, MA
12. Brando B, Barnett D, Janossy G, Mandy F, Autran B, Rothe G et al (2000) Cytofluorometric methods for assessing absolute numbers of cell subsets in blood. Cytometry 42 (6):327–346
13. Wulff S (ed) (2006) Guide to flow cytometry. Dako Cytomation. http://gene-quantification.com/dako-facs-guide.pdf. Accessed 30 May 2017
14. Khan MMT, Pyle BH, Camper AK (2010) Specific and rapid enumeration of viable but nonculturable and viable-culturable gram-negative bacteria by using flow cytometry. Appl Environ Microbiol 76(15):5088–5096

Part V

Streptococcus pneumoniae-Host Interactions: In Vitro and In Vivo Models

Chapter 12

In Vitro Adhesion, Invasion, and Transcytosis of *Streptococcus pneumoniae* with Host Cells

Terry Brissac and Carlos J. Orihuela

Abstract

Physical interactions of bacteria with host cells are often a principal aspect of bacterial pathogenesis. In the case of *Streptococcus pneumoniae* (*Spn*), which does not produce a secreted toxin, adhesion to and/or invasion of host cells is necessary for colonization of the nasopharynx and subsequently to cause opportunistic disease in its human host. Knowledge of how pneumococci interact with host cells thereby helps to explain its biology and may identify potential targets for intervention. One of the simplest, yet powerful, assays that can be leveraged to dissect the molecular basis of this vital host–pathogen interaction is the in vitro adhesion and invasion assay. Among many key results, this assay has been used to discover the bacterial and host determinants involved in bacterial attachment, identify host signaling networks required for uptake of the bacteria into an endosome, and the characterization of the intracellular trafficking machinery that is subverted by *Spn* during development of bacteremia and meningitis. These assays have also been used to characterize the epithelial, endothelial, and/or immune cell response to these bacteria, and to learn how pneumococci disperse from an established biofilm to a planktonic phenotype to colonize another niche and/or transmit. Herein, we will review this protocol, highlighting how simple changes in the bacterial strain or host cell line can elucidate the underlying molecular mechanisms for *Spn* virulence.

Key words Adhesion, Invasion, Translocation, Gentamycin protection assay

1 Introduction

Whether commensal or pathogens, host-associated bacteria physically interact with the latter. In the case of commensals, this ideally allows the development of a mutually beneficial interaction. In the case of pathogenic bacteria, whether opportunistic or not, the same act of colonization can lead to development of disease. As physical interaction is pivotal for the development and the process of infection, it is not surprising that studies on pathogenesis are often focused on the molecular mechanisms responsible for bacterial adherence to the host cell. Other common foci include host receptors and cell signaling involved in cell surface remodeling and bacterial uptake after attachment, the outcome of such interactions, including cell death, bacterial death, or bacterial translocation to

Federico Iovino (ed.), *Streptococcus pneumoniae: Methods and Protocols*, Methods in Molecular Biology, vol. 1968,
https://doi.org/10.1007/978-1-4939-9199-0_12,

the basolateral surface or the adjacent cell. Thus, knowledge gained from the study of bacterial adhesion and invasion is fundamental to our understanding of pathogenesis. Targeting the mechanism (s) involved could potentially be used to subvert the disease process in a therapeutic or prophylactic manner. Along such lines, perhaps the most frequently used assays to examine these interactions is the in vitro adhesion/invasion assay. This is in large part due to its simplicity, low cost, and the rapidness with which the assay can be performed. In its most simple form, this assay consists only of mixing bacteria with a host cell line, washing unattached bacteria away, and observing the outcome of this interaction. This assay is extremely powerful as it can easily be modified or associated with other technologies to test specific molecular interactions.

Streptococcus pneumoniae (*Spn*) pathogenesis is a prime example of the multiple interactions a pathogen can have with a variety of host cell types during the disease process. Most of these interactions can be studied using the adhesion/invasion assay. As a commensal of the human upper respiratory tract (URT), *Spn* colonizes the latter and forms biofilms on the surface of nasopharyngeal epithelium. Aspirated *Spn* in the airway is able to attach and invade epithelial cells, and in severe disease cases the bacterium is able to translocate across the alveolar–capillary barrier and enter the bloodstream to cause invasive pneumococcal disease (IPD). Once in the blood, the bacteria can multiply, and in rare but potentially devastating circumstances the bacteria translocate across the vascular endothelium and gain access to other sites such as the central nervous system and the myocardium. Therefore, deciphering how *Spn* interacts with these different cell types may and lead to strategies that reduce the incidence of pneumococcal diseases.

Some pertinent examples of key findings made with adhesion and invasion assays include the following:

1. *Role of neuraminidase on Spn adhesion to mucosal epithelial cells* [1]. The importance of sialidases (i.e., *nanA*) in *Spn* attachment to epithelial cells was assayed by adhesion assay using isogenic deficient mutants of *Spn*. Pretreatment of cells with neuraminidase inhibitors prior to bacterial addition demonstrated their importance in adhesion. Pretreatment of cells with recombinant neuraminidase was shown to complement the isogenic mutant and to restore *Spn* adhesion.
2. *Biofilm virulence and dispersal on epithelial cells* [2, 3]. Virulence of bacteria from biofilms and the host signals involved in biofilm dispersal were determined. Bacteria grown in planktonic or biofilm conditions were used to infect cells and determine the relative adhesion and virulence of bacteria forming biofilms. Superinfections of cells colonized by *Spn* biofilms using Influenza A virus allowed the identification of host-derived signals (ATP, temperature change, glucose) that induced dispersion of

Spn within biofilms and the release of more virulent planktonic pneumococci capable of transmission.

3. *Polymeric immunoglobulin receptor (pIgR)-mediated uptake in lung epithelial cells* [4]. The mechanisms by which *Spn* is taken up by bronchial epithelial cells and translocate to the basolateral surface was discovered. pIgR was identified as interacting with the adhesin Choline binding protein A (CbpA). Adhesion and invasion experiments in the presence of neutralizing antibody against pIgR or experiments using an isogenic CbpA-deficient mutant confirmed the importance of this interaction in uptake process. Transmigration assays using monolayers grown on Transwell® determined that the deletion of *cbpA* or the neutralization of pIgR inhibited translocation of *Spn* to the basolateral surface suggesting that the bacteria use the pIgR machinery to reach the basolateral surface and possibly gain access to the circulation.
4. *Bacterial translocation across the vascular endothelial cells in the blood–brain barrier to cause meningitis* [5, 6]. Using vascular endothelial cells, Transwell®, electron and fluorescent microscopy, and host cells transfected with dominant negative mutants, host cell signaling triggered upon bacterial interaction and necessary for the uptake and trafficking of *Spn* within endosomes has been learned: after internalization, *Spn* is subject to three fates: (1) being killed within the cell, (2) translocating across the cell layer, and (3) being recycled to the apical surface. Using phase variants of *Spn*, bacterial phase variation has been shown to determine fate in translocation and impact of platelet activating factor receptor (PAFr)-mediated transcytosis or recycling. Immunofluorescence of infected cells determined that bacteria after interaction with PAFr activate beta-arrestin 1 signaling, triggering internalization and trafficking through the canonical Rab-associated endocytosis.
5. *Bacteria-cell interaction during cardiac microlesions formation* [7]. Mouse cardiomyocytes were infected with isogenic mutant bacteria to demonstrate the importance of pneumolysin toxin and H_2O_2 production in *Spn*-mediated cytotoxicity following bacterial uptake by these cells. Invasion assays using endocytotic pathways inhibitors demonstrated that *Spn* invasion occurs through clathrin-mediated endocytosis. The use of neutralizing antibody against both PAFr and pIgR demonstrated that *Spn*-cardiomyocytes interaction occurs independently of the canonical pathways.
6. *Attenuated host response in macrophage isolated from aged mice* [8]. Age-related defects that contribute to the susceptibility of the elderly to pneumonia such as poor Toll-like receptor function, suppressed cytokine production, and reduced phagocytic

killing were assessed. Alveolar macrophages isolated from young and aged mice were exposed to *Spn* ex vivo. Macrophage lysates were used to measure cell activation/cytokines production by ELISA or western-blot analysis.

7. *Determining that lung epithelial cells undergo necroptosis following exposure to Spn* [9]. Using diverse chemical inhibitors, siRNA, and CRISPR/Cas9 gene edited cell lines, the impact of necroptosis signaling and the molecular mechanisms by which pneumolysin kills cells at sublytic concentrations were determined. Supernatants or cell lysates were then used to measure released lactate dehydrogenase (cytotoxicity assay) or to detect phosphorylation of MLKL, the final effector of necroptosis, by phosphor immunoblot, respectively.

Thus, as described above, the assays detailed below are highly amenable to modification in highly specific manner. Undoubtedly, this assay has contributed to our understanding of how *Spn* causes disease.

2 Materials

2.1 Cell Culture

1. Cell line of interest (*see* **Note 1**).
2. Appropriate cell culture media (*see* **Note 2**).
3. 0.05% trypsin–0.02% EDTA (*see* **Note 3**).
4. Multiwell tissue culture plates.
5. Transwell® cell culture inserts (*see* **Note 4**, Fig. 1).
6. Cell counter/hematocytometer.

2.2 Bacterial Culture

1. Blood agar plates: Tryptic soy broth (30 g) supplemented with 1.5% Bacto agar is dissolved in 1 L of distilled water and autoclaved at 121 °C for 30 min. Media is cooled down to 50–55 °C before addition of 5% defibrinated sheep blood. (Media base can be stored in 55 °C water bath without blood for long-term storage.) If deemed necessary, antibiotics can be added prior to pouring the plates.
2. Growth medium, THY: Todd-Hewitt broth (15 g) supplemented with 0.5% yeast extract is dissolved in 500 mL of distilled water and autoclaved at 121 °C for 30 min.
3. *Streptococcus pneumoniae* strain of interest.
4. Spectrophotometer measuring optical density at 621 nm.

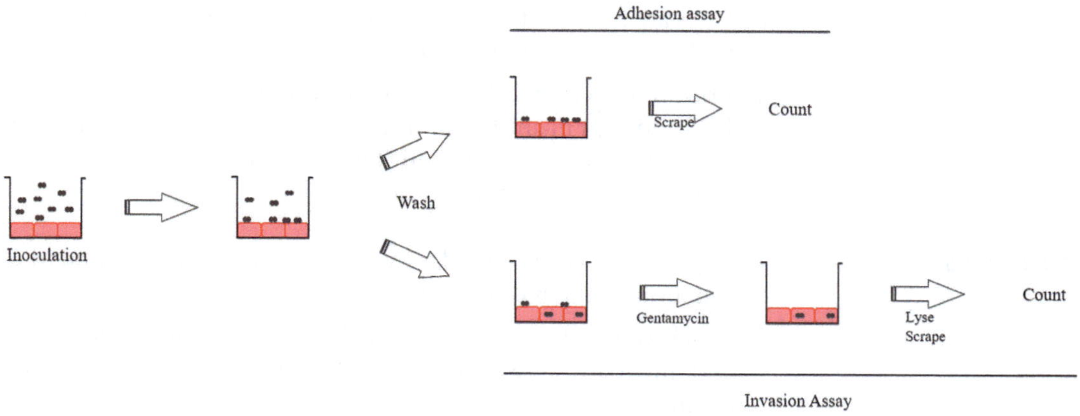

Fig. 1 CFU-based assay setup. Schematic depicting adhesion and invasion assays

2.3 Immuno-fluorescence

1. Coverslips (*see* **Note 5**).
2. 10× phosphate buffered solution (PBS): Mix 80 g of sodium chloride (NaCl), 2 g of potassium chloride (KCl), 14.4 g of disodium phosphate (Na_2HPO_4), and 2.4 g of monopotassium phosphate (KH_2PO4) with 800 mL of distilled water. Adjust pH to 7.4 complete to 1 L and autoclave.
3. Blocking buffer: 1× phosphate buffered solution (PBS) + 1% bovine serum albumin (BSA) + 0.1% Tween 20.
4. Permeabilization buffer: 1× PBS + 0.2% TritonX-100.
5. Washing buffer (PBST): 1× PBS + 0.1% Tween20.
6. Antibodies (*see* **Note 6**).

3 Methods

3.1 Assays Preparation

3.1.1 Bacterial Inoculum Preparation

1. Streak bacteria of interest on BAP overnight at 37 °C and 5% CO_2.
2. Resuspend fresh bacteria in THY at $OD_{621\ nm} = 0.02–0.05$ and grow until $OD_{621\ nm} = 0.3–0.4$ (*see* **Note 7**).
3. Spin down bacteria (3000 × *g* for 10 min) and resuspend in prewarmed DMEM.
4. Measure optical density ($OD_{621\ nm}$) to determine bacterial count and prepare the inoculum accordingly.

3.1.2 Cells Matrix Preparation

1. Detach cells from tissue culture flasks using trypsin–EDTA for 15 min at 37 °C with 5% CO_2.
2. Cells are then spun down (300 × *g* for 5 min) and resuspended in fresh prewarmed media before count determination using cell counter or hematocytometer.

3. Cells are seeded at the appropriate density and incubated overnight at 37 °C and 5% CO_2.
4. Prior to infection, cells are washed twice with prewarmed sterile PBS and kept in antibiotic-free cell culture media. Alternatively, cells can also be seeded in antibiotic-free cell culture media and directly infected the day after.

3.1.3 Infection

1. Replace cell culture media by bacterial inoculum calibrated in function of the required multiplicity of infection.
2. Synchronize attachment by centrifugation at 300 × *g* for 5 min and incubate at 37 °C/5% CO_2 for the required amount of time.

3.2 CFU Count-Based Assays (Fig. 2)

3.2.1 Adhesion/Associated Assay

1. After 30 min of incubation (*see* **Note 8**) cells are gently washed three times in PBS to eliminate unbound bacteria.
2. Scrape cells in PBS, and cell suspension is serially diluted before plating.
3. Plates are incubated at 37 °C 5% CO_2 overnight before count determination.

3.2.2 Invasion Assay (Gentamycin Protection Assay)

1. After 30 min of incubation, cells are washed three times with PBS and resuspended in fresh prewarmed cell culture media.
2. Incubate for 30 more minutes to maximize invasion of already attached bacteria.
3. Replace culture media by fresh media containing 200 μg/mL of gentamycin to kill extracellular bacteria and incubate plates for 1 h at 37 °C/5% CO_2.
4. Wash wells three times with PBS, resuspend in cold distilled water, and incubate for 20 min at 4 °C (*see* **Note 9**).
5. Scrap the wells and plate; use serial dilution, if necessary, before plating; and incubate overnight at 37 °C 5% CO_2.

3.2.3 Transcytosis Assay (*See* **Note 10**)

The volumes described in this section are used in a 12-well plate setup.

1. After 30 min of incubation, wash both sides of the inserts three times with PBS.
2. Move inserts to a new plate and add 450 μL of media in the upper chamber and 900 μL of media in the lower chamber and incubate for 30 more minutes at 37 °C with 5% CO_2.
3. Add 50 μL of 2 mg/mL of gentamycin in media (final concentration 200 μg/ml, bactericidal concentration) in the upper chamber and 100 μL of 200 μg/mL of gentamycin in media (final concentration 20 μg/ml, bacteriostatic concentration) and incubate for 1 h at 37 °C with 5% CO_2.

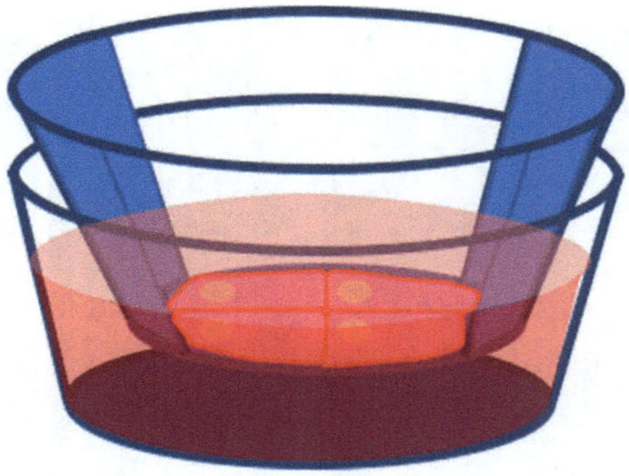

Fig. 2 Transcytosis assay setup. Schematic of the Transwell® inserts used for transcytosis assays

4. Plate 200–400 μL from the lower chamber to determine transcytosis at 1 h.
5. Wash inserts three times with PBS (both sides), move them to a new plate and add media containing bacteriostatic concentration of gentamycin before incubation for 1 h at 37 °C with 5% CO_2.
6. Plate 200–400 μL of both chambers on BAP (*see* **Note 10**).

3.3 Fluorescence-Based Assays

3.3.1 Adhesion Assay

In this assay, staining of the bacteria without permeabilization of the membrane allows only for the detection of adherent bacteria without considering the internalized ones. Adhesion rate can then be determined by counting the number observed after observation of 10–25 fields.

1. At each required timepoint, wash cells three times with PBS and fix for 20 min at RT with 4% PFA in PBS.
2. Wash coverslips once with PBS and quench aldehydes using PBS–NH_4Cl 50 mM for 5 min at 4 °C.
3. Wash once with PBS and incubate in blocking buffer for 1 h at RT.
4. Incubate with anti-*Spn* primary antibody overnight at 4 °C, then wash three times in PBST.
5. Incubate for 1 h with dye-labeled secondary antibody and wash three times in PBST.
6. Counterstain with DAPI and mount in FluorSave (Millipore) before observation.

3.3.2 Invasion Assay (Fig. 3)

In this assay, bacteria are stained twice before and after permeabilization of the membrane. Extracellular bacteria will appear stained by both fluorophores while intracellular ones appear stained only once (i.e., with the fluorophore used after permeabilization). Invasion rate

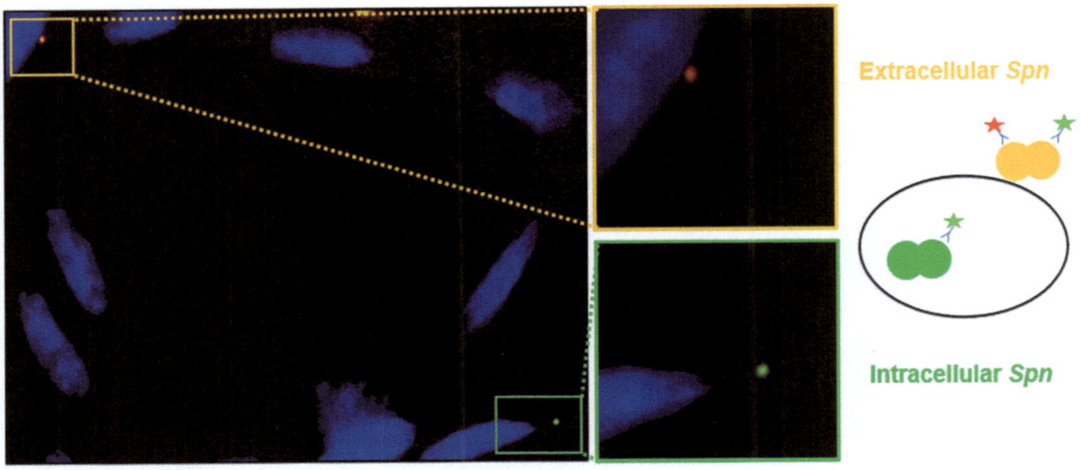

Fig. 3 Fluorescence assay example. Immunofluorescence microscopy on HL-1 cardiomyocytes after 1 h of infection by *Spn*. Pneumococci were stained before (Rhodamine, Red) and after (FITC, green) permeabilization of the cell membrane using anti-serotype 4 antibody. (Adapted from Brissac et al. 2017, Copyright © American Society for Microbiology, IAI 86(1):e00569-17, DOI: https:/doi.org/10.1128/IAI.00569-17, 2017)

can then be determined by counting the number observed after observation of 10–25 fields.

1. Perform **steps 1–5** described in adhesion assay.
2. Permeabilize cells using permeabilization buffer for 10 min at RT.
3. Repeat **steps 4–6** using a secondary antibody labeled with a different dye.
4. Counterstain with DAPI and mount in FluorSave (Millipore) before observation.

4 Notes

1. Multiples cell types/lines can be used (*see* below). Most of the cell lines can be purchased from ATCC (American Type Culture Collection) or from various suppliers (e.g., Sigma-Aldrich and ABM). Endothelial cell lines: HUVEC (human umbilical vein endothelial cells), hCMEC/D3 (human blood–brain barrier). Epithelial cell lines: A549 (mouse lung epithelial), Detroit 562 (human pharyngeal). Immune cells: J774.A1 (mouse macrophages), THP-1 (human macrophages), BMDM (bone-marrow derived macrophages).
2. Appropriate media for each cell line and required supplements are provided by suppliers.

3. Trypsin–EDTA does not allow detachment of all cell types. In these cases, use of gentle scraping using cell scrapers may be necessary.
4. Different pore sizes are available. The latter must be chosen according to the cell line used to allow bacterial but not eukaryotic cell passage.
5. Chamber slides can also be used, allowing for multiple washes and ready-to-observe slides.
6. Serotype-specific anti-*Spn* serum can be purchased from Statens Institute. If available, fluorescent *Spn* or FITC-conjugated bacteria can also be used.
7. Culture of some bacterial strains growing faster than others (e.g., noncapsulated strains) can be started at a different initial $OD_{621\ nm}$ reaching mid-log phase at the same time.
8. Timing of initial interaction/adhesion can be extended. However, longer exposure time increases the probability of internalization of bacteria, intracellular killing, and/or release of the bacteria associated with "reinternalization" events.
9. Cells can also be lysed using 1× PBS–0.1% Triton X-100 in order to release internalized bacteria.
10. To attest the integrity of the cell layer, TEER (Trans Epithelial/Endothelial Resistance) can be measured prior to infection. An Evans Blue post-assay [10, 11] can also be performed: In a new plate, add 1 mL of media in both chambers before addition of 25 μL of 0.5% Evans Blue in the upper chamber and incubation for 1 h at 37 °C. Add extra wells with 0, 0.5, 1, or 15 μL of Evans Blue as a standard. Measure absorbance at 620 nm for wells from both chambers. Only wells presenting absorbance lower than the 0.5 μL control should be kept for analysis.

References

1. Brittan JL, Buckeridge TJ, Finn A, Kadioglu A, Jenkinson HF (2012) Pneumococcal neuraminidase A: an essential upper airway colonization factor for Streptococcus pneumoniae. Mol Oral Microbiol 27:270–283
2. Marks LR, Davidson BA, Knight PR, Hakansson AP (2013) Interkingdom signaling induces Streptococcus pneumoniae biofilm dispersion and transition from asymptomatic colonization to disease. MBio 4:e00438–e00413
3. Sanchez CJ, Kumar N, Lizcano A, Shivshankar P, Dunning Hotopp JC, Jorgensen JH, Tettelin H, Orihuela CJ (2011) Streptococcus pneumoniae in biofilms are unable to cause invasive disease due to altered virulence determinant production. PLoS One 6:e28738
4. Zhang JR, Mostov KE, Lamm ME, Nanno M, Shimida S, Ohwaki M, Tuomanen E (2000) The polymeric immunoglobulin receptor translocates pneumococci across human nasopharyngeal epithelial cells. Cell 102:827–837
5. Radin JN, Orihuela CJ, Murti G, Guglielmo C, Murray PJ, Tuomanen EI (2005) Beta-Arrestin 1 participates in platelet-activating factor receptor-mediated endocytosis of streptococcus pneumoniae. Infect Immun 73:7827–7835

6. Ring A, Weiser JN, Tuomanen EI (1998) Pneumococcal trafficking across the blood-brain barrier. Molecular analysis of a novel bidirectional pathway. J Clin Invest 102:347–360
7. Brissac T, Shenoy AT, Patterson LA, Orihuela CJ (2017) Cell invasion and pyruvate oxidase derived H2O2 are critical for Streptococcus pneumoniae mediated cardiomyocyte killing. Infect Immun. https://doi.org/10.1128/IAI.00569-17
8. Hinojosa CA, Akula Suresh Babu R, Rahman MM, Fernandes G, Boyd AR, Orihuela CJ (2014) Elevated A20 contributes to age-dependent macrophage dysfunction in the lungs. Exp Gerontol 54:58–66
9. Gonzalez-Juarbe N, Bradley KM, Shenoy AT, Gilley RP, Reyes LF, Hinojosa CA, Restrepo MI, Dube PH, Bergman MA, Orihuela CJ (2017) Pore-forming toxin-mediated ion dysregulation leads to death receptor-independent necroptosis of lung epithelial cells during bacterial pneumonia. Cell Death Differ 24:917–928
10. Radu M, Chernoff J (2013) An in vivo assay to test blood vessel permeability. J Vis Exp. https://doi.org/10.3791/50062:e50062
11. Nguyen S, Baker K, Padman BS, Patwa R, Dunstan RA, Weston TA, Schlosser K, Bailey B, Lithgow T, Lazarou M, Luque A, Rohwer F, Blumberg RS, Barr JJ (2017) Bacteriophage transcytosis provides a mechanism to cross epithelial cell layers. MBio 8: e01874–e01817

Chapter 13

Growing and Characterizing Biofilms Formed by *Streptococcus pneumoniae*

Yashuan Chao, Caroline Bergenfelz, and Anders P. Hakansson

Abstract

It is estimated that over 80% of bacterial infections are associated with biofilm formation. Biofilms are organized bacterial communities formed on abiotic surfaces, such as implanted or inserted medical devices, or on biological surfaces, such as epithelial linings and mucosal surfaces. Biofilm growth is advantageous for the bacterial organism as it protects the bacteria from antimicrobial host factors and allows the bacteria to reside in the host without causing excessive inflammation. Like many other opportunistic pathogens of the respiratory tract, *Streptococcus pneumoniae* forms biofilms during asymptomatic carriage, which promotes, among other things, persistence in the niche, intraspecies and interspecies communication, and spread of bacterial DNA. Changes within the colonizing environment resulting from host assaults, such as virus infection, can induce biofilm dispersion where bacteria leave the biofilm and disseminate to other sites with ensuing infection. In this chapter, we present methodology to form complex biofilms in the nasopharynx of mice and to evaluate the biofilm structure and function in this environment. Furthermore, we present methods that recapitulate this biofilm phenotype in vitro by incorporating crucial factors associated with the host environment and describe how these models can be used to study biofilm function, transformation, and dispersion.

Key words Biofilm, *Streptococcus pneumoniae*, Respiratory tract, Nasopharynx, Epithelium, Mucosa, Carriage, Colonization, Transformation, Competence, Dispersion, Virulence

1 Introduction

Biofilms are complex communities of aggregated microbes, often comprising multiple species, encased in a self-produced, three-dimensional polymeric matrix consisting of polysaccharides, lipids, proteins, and nucleic acids. The matrix has both structural and protective properties and often incorporates host structures that improves the "stealth" and survival of the bacterial community. Production of matrix exopolysaccharide is known both to affect the adhesion to host surfaces and to protect against the host immune system [1, 2]. The presence of extracellular DNA (eDNA) and DNA-binding proteins serves as a scaffold on which the biofilm is formed [3, 4]. eDNA is also used as a substrate for

Federico Iovino (ed.), *Streptococcus pneumoniae: Methods and Protocols*, Methods in Molecular Biology, vol. 1968,
https://doi.org/10.1007/978-1-4939-9199-0_13,

genetic transformation and spread of fitness traits, such as antibiotic resistance [5, 6]. The structure of the biofilm and the specialization of bacteria, with distinct metabolism and gene expression profiles, provide advantages for biofilm persistence in the host niche through increased resistance to environmental and host challenges [7–9].

It is estimated that approximately 65–80% of infections are associated with microbial biofilms [7, 10]. However, the contribution of biofilms to disease varies between species. Biofilms are directly required to cause some infections, such as dental caries, and are a common feature during chronic infection, but are often associated with asymptomatic carriage of opportunistic pathogens on our mucosal linings or with bacterial growth on medical devices. Together, this suggests that biofilms sometimes directly cause disease but more commonly act as a dormant reservoir of pathogenic organisms [11, 12]. This is supported by the fact that biofilm bacteria, in most cases, are less virulent than their planktonically growing counterparts [13, 14]. Yet, as biofilms persist and survive better at the site of infection, they can seed off virulent organisms under certain circumstances [14]. As biofilm bacteria also survive better on surfaces outside the body [15, 16], they contribute significantly to bacterial spread in daycare and hospital settings [17, 18].

In this chapter, we will present methods used to form, assess, and functionally evaluate biofilms formed by the opportunistic respiratory pathogen *Streptococcus pneumoniae* (the pneumococcus). This is an updated and extended version of a prior methods chapter [19] and focuses only on pneumococcal biofilms. *S. pneumoniae* effectively colonizes the mucosal surface of the nasopharynx to the extent that it is estimated that close to half the world's population is colonized at any given time [20]. That pneumococci form biofilms during colonization in vivo was first suggested indirectly in the late 1990s, as it is more difficult to eradicate colonization than infection. This is in agreement with the increased resistance of biofilms to antimicrobial agents [21, 22]. Work from our laboratory has confirmed these observations in a colonization model in mice [23]. Figure 1a shows a representative scanning electron micrograph of a pneumococcal biofilm in vivo. Pneumococcal biofilms have also been detected in patients with otitis media and chronic sinusitis [24–27] as well as in animal models, where the biofilms act as a reservoir for the release of pathogenic organisms [12]. Furthermore, biofilms constitute the main life form of the pneumococcus during colonization of the nasopharynx [23, 28–31].

Various virulence factors have been implicated in biofilm formation in vitro using model systems primarily conducted on abiotic surfaces [32–35]. Additionally, pneumococcal biofilm bacteria display an altered virulence gene expression leading to a decreased

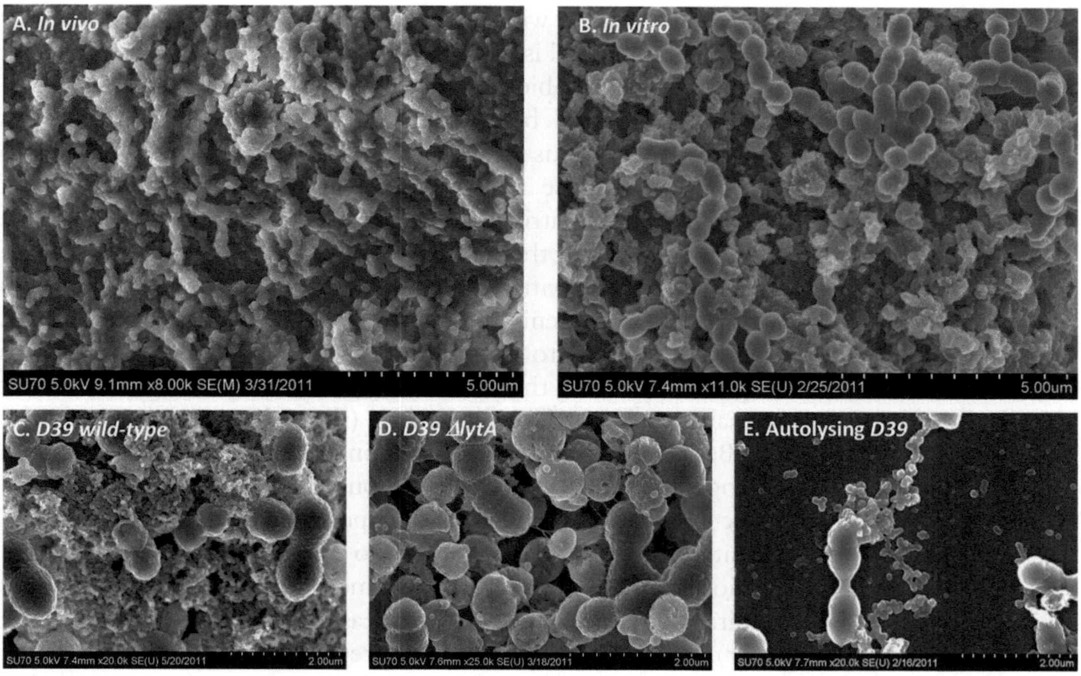

Fig. 1 Pneumococcal biofilms formed in the nasopharynx of a BALB/c mouse (**a**) or on bronchial epithelial cells (**b**). Both biofilms show aggregation and organization of bacteria (diplococci and small chains) into clusters with empty spaces that will develop into pores, and the formation of extracellular matrix encasing the bacteria. The matrix appears to originate from lysed cells, as early biofilms of D39 wild-type bacteria have high levels of matrix encasing the bacterial cells (**c**) whereas the isogenic mutant lacking the major autolysin, LytA, is devoid of matrix (**d**). The smaller spheres in image (**d**) potentially depict extracellular vesicles. To show that the morphology of the debris after cell lysis is similar to the morphology of the extracellular matrix, image (**e**) depicts remnants from pneumococci lysing after treatment with a human milk protein complex HAMLET

virulence of biofilm bacteria in vivo [13, 36, 37]. However, until recently, in vitro studies did not take the host environment into consideration.

The methods described here incorporate key features of the nasopharyngeal environment necessary to obtain biofilms in vitro that are structurally and functionally equivalent to colonizing biofilms in vivo [23, 31] (*see* Fig. 1b for a representative example). Such key features include temperature, the substratum, nutrient availability, and the duration of biofilm formation. Growth at a temperature of approximately 34 °C is consistent with that measured in the nasopharynx of humans and mice [38] while growth on a respiratory epithelial substratum provides relevant interactions with host tissue. These aspects, in combination with growth in nutrient-limiting media over at least 48 h, were necessary for optimal biofilm formation, which is consistent with the high bacterial density and nutritional starvation typical of biofilms in general [39]. By employing these key features of the nasopharyngeal environment, we obtained well-structured biofilms encased in extracellular matrix with high tolerance to antibiotic treatment for most pneumococcal isolates tested, a phenotype not observed with biofilms grown on abiotic surfaces, such as glass or plastic [23]. Furthermore, bacterial burden and antibiotic resistance of biofilms produced by various strains correlated well with their ability to colonize the mouse nasopharynx. Interestingly, the majority of the extracellular matrix in pneumococcal biofilms appear to derive from lysing cells in the biofilm (Fig. 1c–e). The matrix of mature pneumococcal in vitro biofilms (Fig. 1c), but not of biofilms formed by an isogenic mutant lacking the major autolysin LytA (Fig. 1d), is similar to the morphology of lysing pneumococcal cells (Fig. 1e). In fact, the biofilms formed by the isogenic mutant appear completely devoid of matrix (Fig. 1d).

Based on the studies so far, this in vitro model can act as a useful surrogate model for in vivo colonization, in which functional aspects can be determined. Such aspects include colonization propensity, genetic transformation [5, 6], and biofilm dispersion. Dispersion can be induced by common disease triggers, such as respiratory viruses [40–42], increased temperature (mimicking fever), or ATP or norepinephrine (representing damage-associated molecular patterns; DAMPs [14]). Furthermore, the bacterial phenotypes can be verified using RNA-sequencing or quantitative reverse-transcriptase PCR (qRT-PCR) [43]. The models described in this chapter can serve as a surrogate model for studies related to the colonization state of pneumococci in humans as well as a model to study the mechanisms of transition to disease.

2 Materials

2.1 Preparation of Bacterial Strains

1. Pneumococcal strains of interest.
2. Bacterial growth medium: Prepare Todd-Hewitt medium according to the manufacturer's instructions and supplement with 0.5% yeast extract (THY; BD Bioscience). Sterilize the medium either by autoclavation or sterile filtration using a 0.45 μm vacuum filter system.
3. Spectrophotometer for measuring optical density at 600 nm (OD_{600}) (*see* **Note 1**).
4. Bacterial freezing solution: Prepare 80% (v/v) glycerol in water and sterilize the solution by autoclavation (*see* **Note 2**).
5. Blood agar plates: Blood agar plates can be purchased from a vendor, but can also be made in the laboratory. For preparation of blood agar plates, prepare tryptic soy agar according to the manufacturer's instructions and supplement with 5% sheep blood. For step-by-step preparation of blood agar plates (*see* **Note 3**).

2.2 Preparation of the Epithelial Substratum

1. Cells: Use epithelial cell lines, such as human mucoepidermoid pulmonary carcinoma cells NCI-H292 (CRL-1849, ATCC) or human lung carcinoma cells A549 (CCL-185, ATCC). Other cell types can be used (*see* **Note 4**).
2. Cell culture medium: Supplement RPMI-1640 medium (containing 0.3 mg/ml of L-glutamine) with 10% fetal bovine serum, 1 mM sodium pyruvate, 100 U/ml penicillin, and 100 μg/ml streptomycin.
3. Cell detachment: Prepare phosphate-buffered saline (PBS; 0.4 M NaCl, 0.0027 M KCl, 0.010 M phosphate buffer, pH 7.2; Medicago) for washing the cell monolayer. Use trypsin (0.25%) in PBS (pH 7.2) for detachment of cells (can be purchased ready-made from various vendors).
4. Cell fixation: Prepare 4% (w/v) paraformaldehyde (PFA) solution in PBS.

2.3 Biofilm Formation In Vitro on Fixed Epithelial Cells

1. 24-well plates with a substratum of PFA-fixed epithelial cells (from Subheading 3.1.2).
2. Wash solution: Use PBS, pH 7.2 (*see* Subheading 2.2).
3. Frozen stock(s) of pneumococci (from Subheading 3.1.1).
4. Chemically defined medium (CDM): Prepare CDM from reagent stocks (*see* **Note 5** and Table 1 for full details) including supplementing the medium with 1 g/l choline chloride, 0.75 g/l L-cysteine hydrochloride, and 2.5 g/l of sodium bicarbonate. Filter-sterilize with a 0.45 μm vacuum filter system.
5. Incubator system set to 34 °C and 5% CO_2 for biofilm growth.

2.4 Biofilm Formation In Vitro on Live Epithelial Cells

1. 24-well plate with live, confluent epithelial cells (from Subheading 3.1.2).
2. Mature pneumococcal biofilms (from Subheading 3.1.3).
3. Antibiotic-free cell culture medium: Supplement RPMI-1640 medium (containing 0.3 mg/ml L-glutamine) with 2% fetal bovine serum and 1 mM sodium pyruvate.

2.5 Biofilm Dispersal with Heat In Vitro

1. Mature pneumococcal biofilms (from Subheading 3.1.3).
2. Chemically defined media (CDM) (*see* Table 1 and **Note 5**)
3. A separate incubator set at 38.5 °C.
4. Blood agar plates (*see* Subheading 2.1).

2.6 Biofilm Formation In Vivo

1. Frozen stock of pneumococci (from Subheading 3.1.1).
2. Wash and re-suspension buffer: Use PBS, pH 7.2 (*see* Subheading 2.2).
3. BALB/cByJ mice, 6–8 weeks old (*see* **Note 6**).

Table 1
Preparation of CDM

Ingredients for stock solutions			
Stock A in water[a]		***Stock C*** in water[a]	
Magnesium sulfate, heptahydrate	7000	DL-Alanine	1000
Manganese sulfate, anhydrous	50	L-Arginine, free base	1000
Ferrous sulfate, heptahydrate	50	Glycine	1000
Ferric nitrate, nonahydrate	10	Hydroxy-L-Proline	1000
Calcium chloride, anhydrous	51	L-Isoleucine	1000
Stock B in 1 M HCl[a]		L-Lysine	1000
L-Aspartic acid	1000	L-Proline	1000
L-Cysteine, free base	5000	L-Serine	1000
L-Cystine dihydrochloride	500	L-Threonine	2000
L-Glutamic acid	1000	L-Valine	1000
L-Glutamine	2000	***Stock D*** in 1 M HCl[a]	
L-Histidine, free base	1000	Adenine, free base	200
L-Leucine	1000	***Stock E*** in 1 M NaOH[a]	
L-Methionine	1000	Guanine hydrochloride	200
L-Phenylalanine	1000	Uracil	200
L-Tryptophan	1000	Folic acid	8
L-Tyrosine, free base	1000		
Stock F in water[a]			
PABA	2	Pyridoxal hydrochloride	10
Biotin	2	Pyridoxamine dihydrochloride	10
Niacinamide	10	Riboflavin	20
β-Nicotinamide adenine dinucleotide	25	Thiamine hydrochloride	10
D-Calcium pantothenate	20	Cyanocobalamin	1

[a]Quantities are in mg (*see* **Note 5** for details).

Ingredients for preparation of 1 liter of CDM[b, c]			
Sodium acetate, trihydrate	4500	Stocks A–E	1 aliquot
Sodium phosphate, monobasic, monohydrate	3195	Glucose	10,000
Sodium phosphate, dibasic, anhydrous	7350	Choline chloride	1000
Potassium phosphate, monobasic	1000	L-Cysteine hydrochloride	750
Potassium phosphate, dibasic	200	Sodium bicarbonate	5000

[b]Quantities are in mg.
[c]Per 50-ml aliquot, add 1 ml of freshly thawed Stock F to make the medium complete.

2.7 Biomass and Antibiotic Resistance of In Vitro Biofilms

1. Gentamicin solution (50 mg/ml).
2. Use PBS, pH 7.2, for serial dislutions (see Subheading 2.2).
3. Use blood agar plates for viable plate counts (*see* Subheading 2.1).

2.8 Biomass Determination of In Vivo Biofilms

1. 70% (v/v) ethanol in water, in a plastic squeeze bottle.
2. Dissection equipment: scissors, forceps, curved tweezers, and homogenization bags.
3. Use PBS, pH 7.2, for serial dilutions (*see* Subheading 2.2).
4. Use blood agar plates for viable plate counts (*see* Subheading 2.1).

2.9 Transformation Efficiency of Biofilms

1. Use blood agar plates (*see* Subheading 2.1) without antibiotics or with antibiotics at concentrations corresponding to the antibiotic resistance markers in the pneumococcal strains used.

2.10 Scanning Electron Microscopy (SEM)

1. Fixation solution: Prepare 2.5% glutaraldehyde, 0.075% ruthenium red, and 0.075 M lysine acetate (*see* **Note 7**) in 0.1 M sodium cacodylate buffer (pH 7.2).
2. Wash solution: Prepare 0.075% ruthenium red in 0.2 M sodium cacodylate buffer (pH 7.2).
3. Ethanol solutions ranging from 50% (v/v) in water to absolute ethanol with 10% interval increases.
4. Critical point dryer.
5. Glass cover slips for cell growth, SEM stubs and sputter coater.

2.11 RNA Isolation and qRT-PCR of In Vitro Biofilms

1. Cell wall-degrading solution: Add 1 mg/ml lysozyme and 50 U/ml mutanolysin to TE buffer (Tris–EDTA; 10 mM Tris–HCl, 1 mM EDTA, pH 8.0).
2. Lysis solutions: Prepare 1% (w/v) sodium dodecyl sulfate (SDS) stock in water. TRI Reagent solution (or similar).
3. RNA purification: Zymo Research Direct-zol™ RNA Mini-Prep Kit (*see* **Note 8**).
4. DNA digestion: DNase I and 10× DNase I buffer (Thermo Fisher Scientific).
5. Phenol–chloroform–isoamyl alcohol separation: Phenol–chloroform–isoamyl alcohol mixture (49.5:49.5:1 ratio v/v/v; Sigma), 3 M sodium acetate, and absolute ethanol.
6. Spectrophotometer for UV absorbance readings (*see* **Note 9**).
7. Gel electrophoresis: Gibco-Agarose (Invitrogen), TAE buffer (per liter: 4.84 g Tris base, 1.14 ml glacial acetic acid, and 2 ml of 0.5 M EDTA solution at pH 8.0, in water), and gel electrophoresis system.

Table 2
Primers for qRT-PCR

Primer sequences for qRT-PCR gene expression analysis		
Gene	**Forward (5′ → 3′)**	**Reverse (5′ → 3′)**
cps2	CGTGATGCAGATGTAGTAATTGCG	TGTAAGTGGCAAGCGATACGATGC
comD	GGTTCGTATCATGAGCGTTT	CCTGAAGGAGTCATCGTCAT
gyrA	ATGGTCTCAAAGCGCTGAAT	TGGCGATACGACTCATACCA
licD2	ACGAGCAGTTCACGGTGATAGCAA	ATCCCTTCCTTACCGATCCCAACT
lytA	GGCTGGCAGAAGAATGACACTG	GCCGTCTGTGTGCTTCCT

8. cDNA synthesis: iScript™ cDNA synthesis kit (Bio-Rad).
9. qRT-PCR: Primer pairs for genes of interest (*see* **Note 10** and Table 2) and iQ™ SYBR Green Supermix (Bio-Rad).

3 Methods

3.1 Biofilm Formation In Vitro

Cells from the respiratory tract generally provide a better surface for pneumococcal biofilm formation than cells from other parts of the body (such as keratinocytes and sarcoma cells; Hakansson AP, unpublished observation). When grown on respiratory epithelial cells, most pneumococcal strains have the capacity to form well-structured and functional biofilms in contrast to the poorly developed biofilms that form on abiotic surfaces over the same time period (unpublished observations; [23]). In general, pneumococcal biofilms are able to form on either fixed or live epithelial cells in our models. However, to enable biofilm formation on live epithelial cells, biofilm bacteria first formed on fixed cells are transferred onto live cells, as these bacteria have a lower expression of cytotoxic factors in comparison with broth-grown, planktonic pneumococci that show considerable toxicity towards live epithelial cells [14, 43]. *See* Fig. 2 for a schematic of the methodologies presented here.

3.1.1 Preparation of Bacterial Strains

1. Streak out the pneumococcal strain(s) of interest on blood agar plates and incubate overnight at 37 °C (*see* **Note 11**).
2. Using a sterile inoculation loop, transfer individual colonies from the blood agar plate into a glass tube (16 × 100 mm) or a 15-ml conical tube containing 10 ml of THY medium. Tighten the cap and grow statically at 37 °C to an OD_{600} of approximately 0.6 (*see* **Note 12**).
3. Add 2 ml of 80% glycerol solution directly to the 10 ml culture, mix well by pipetting, then transfer the bacterial suspension to

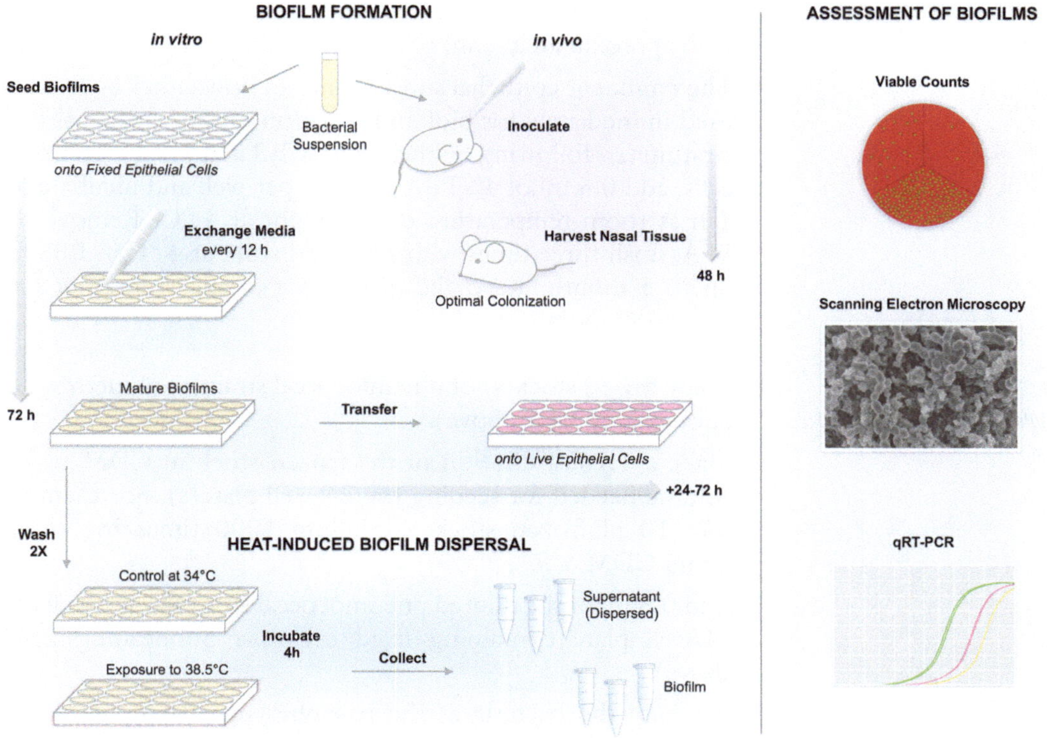

Fig. 2 A cartoon of the methodology presented in this protocol. Pneumococcal biofilms can be formed in vitro on epithelial cells (*see* Subheading 3.1) or in vivo in the mouse nasopharynx (*see* Subheading 3.3). In vitro biofilms are formed on fixed epithelial cells, but mature biofilms can then be transferred and maintained on live epithelial cells (*see* Subheading 3.1). Mature biofilms formed on fixed epithelial cells are also used in biofilm dispersal induced by exposure to increased temperature (mimicking fever), where both the supernatant and biofilm fractions are collected for comparison (*see* Subheading 3.2). Ways to assess the biofilm phenotype (*see* Subheading 3.4) are shown in the right part of the cartoon

microcentrifuge cryotubes in 500 μl aliquots and store at −80 °C (*see* **Note 13**).

3.1.2 Preparation of the Epithelial Substratum

1. Propagate epithelial cell line(s) of choice in cell culture flasks.
2. To passage the cells, remove the medium, wash the cell monolayer twice with PBS to remove residual medium, and detach the confluent cell monolayer from the flask by adding trypsin solution, noting that the detachment time will vary depending on the cell line. Detachment of cells can be visualized macroscopically as well as in a microscope. Resuspend the detached cells in fresh cell culture medium. (The fetal bovine serum contains trypsin inhibitors that will inactivate trypsin to allow reattachment of the cells.) Add 0.5 ml cell suspension per well in 24-well cell culture plates and incubate at 37 °C in 5% CO_2 until near-confluent.

3. Aspirate the medium and wash the cell monolayers three times with approximately 1 ml of PBS per well.
4. The confluent epithelial substratum can now either be fixed or used immediately for biofilm formation on live epithelial substratum (*see* following Subheadings 3.1.3 and 3.1.4). To fix the cells, add 0.5 ml of 4% PFA solution per well and incubate for 1 h at room temperature or overnight at 4 °C. Remove the PFA, wash three times with PBS, and store at 4 °C in PBS for up to a month. Keep the plates in a plastic storage box to prevent evaporation.

3.1.3 Biofilm Formation In Vitro on Fixed Epithelial Cells

1. Thaw frozen stock(s) of pneumococcal strain(s) of interest (*see* Subheading 3.1.1 above).
2. Make a 1:1000 dilution of the frozen stock in CDM to the volume needed for seeding the 24-well plate(s). For example, take 10 μl frozen stock and dilute 1000 times by adding 10 ml CDM.
3. Add 0.5 ml of the diluted pneumococcal stock in each well of a 24-well plate containing fixed cells (*see* Subheading 3.1.2 above).
4. Incubate the bacteria at the nasopharyngeal temperature of 34 °C in 5% CO_2 for optimal biofilm formation (*see* **Note 14**), carefully exchanging the supernatant with 0.5 ml fresh CDM approximately every 12 h (*see* **Note 15** for important details regarding the medium). Avoid disturbing the biofilm as much as possible by keeping the plate leveled, pipetting off the used medium with a 5-ml or 10-ml serological pipette, and adding 0.5 ml fresh CDM slowly down the side of each well (*see* **Note 16**).
5. Grow biofilms for appropriate times, but for at least 48 h, to obtain mature biofilms (*see* **Note 15**).
6. Assess biofilm structure and function according to Subheading 3.4.

3.1.4 Biofilm Formation In Vitro on Live Epithelial Cells

1. Grow live epithelial cells to near confluence as described in Subheading 3.1.2 above.
2. Preparation of live epithelial cells for inoculation with biofilm bacteria formed on fixed epithelial cells: Make sure that the cells have been grown in antibiotic-free media for the last 24 h. Remove the media from the cells and wash the epithelium twice with PBS (*see* **Note 17**).
3. Carefully remove the supernatant from biofilms that have already been grown to maturity on fixed epithelial cells (i.e., for at least 48 h and preferably for 72 h).

4. Gently resuspend the biofilm bacteria in 0.5 ml fresh antibiotic-free cell culture medium (prewarmed to 34 °C) using a 200–1000 μl pipette (*see* **Note 18**).
5. Dilute the resuspended biofilm bacteria from one well approximately 1:5–1:30 in fresh antibiotic-free cell culture medium and transfer 0.5 ml per well to live, confluent epithelial cells.
6. Grow the bacteria on cells at 34 °C in 5% CO_2, taking care to change the antibiotic-free cell culture medium carefully so as not to disturb the attached biofilm bacteria, but at the same time remove non-attached bacteria growing in the media. Also, change media frequently, at least every 4–6 h, to avoid epithelial cell toxicity resulting from overgrowth, production of toxic molecules, and depletion of nutrients in the media by rapidly growing, passively-detached pneumococci (*see* **Note 19**).
7. The pneumococcal biofilm will re-form within 24 h and the epithelial cells should be viable up to 72 h after the transfer (*see* **Note 20**).
8. Assess biofilm structure and function according to Subheading 3.4.

3.2 Biofilm Dispersal In Vitro

Colonization is thought to be the first and necessary step in pneumococcal pathogenesis. While colonizing bacteria primarily reside in the nasopharynx without causing symtoms, changes in the nasopharyngeal environment associated with virus infection and virus-induced signals, such as increased temperature (fever), can induce dispersal of a population from the biofilm that is transcriptionally and phenotypically distinct [14]. For example, virus-dispersed or heat-dispersed bacteria have major alterations in virulence gene expression, resulting in a more inflammatory and more invasive bacterial population than the biofilms they came from or compared with broth-grown planktonic bacteria [43]. Understanding biofilm dispersal and the transition to disease offers opportunities to target pneumococcal disease rather than asymptomatic colonization. The methods below describe biofilm dispersal in response to heat exposure (mimicking fever). Other dispersal signals have been identified [14] and can be used in the same system and evaluated in the same way.

3.2.1 Dispersion of Pneumococcal Biofilms with Heat

1. Prepare biofilms in vitro for 48–72 h according to Subheading 3.1.3 in two 24-well plates.
2. Carefully remove the supernatant, wash twice with 0.5 ml CDM, and replace with 0.5 ml fresh CDM by slowly adding it down the side of the well.
3. For heat-induced dispersal, place one plate in an incubator set to febrile-range temperature (38.5 °C) and keep a control plate at 34 °C during the incubation time. For biofilm dispersal with

other reagents, incubate mature biofilms with and without the reagents at appropriate concentrations and incubate for up to 4 h before assessing dispersal of the biofilm.

4. After 4 h of incubation, transfer the supernatant from treated and untreated biofilms with a 5-ml or 10-ml serological pipette into pre-labeled microcentrifuge tubes and vortex the tubes. Resuspend the remaining biofilm in 0.5 ml PBS and then determine the total viable counts for all samples according to Subheading 3.4.1 and/or save the bacteria for gene expression analysis according to Subheading 3.4.5 below.
5. Biofilm dispersal can be determined either as the increased number of bacterial colonies observed in the supernatant of treated biofilms or as a ratio of supernatant over biofilm biomass for each sample. In the latter example, the ratio should increase with increased dispersal as a result of release of biofilm bacteria into the supernatant.

3.3 Biofilm Formation In Vivo

S. pneumoniae is an efficient colonizer of the nasopharyngeal mucosal surfaces. Although the pneumococcus is an almost exclusively human pathogen, mouse models of colonization have been established that mimic the majority of the phenotypes of colonization observed in man [44, 45]. To induce bacterial carriage and assess biofilm colonization burden, the methods described below will best reproduce human colonization [23, 44].

3.3.1 Colonization of the Mouse Nasopharynx

1. Thaw frozen stock(s) of pneumococcal strain(s) of interest to study with known CFU concentrations (*see* **Note 21**).
2. Pellet the pneumococci by centrifugation at 9,000 × *g* for 2 min in a microcentrifuge and discard the supernatant. Wash the bacterial pellet in PBS twice. Resuspend the final pellet in PBS to a concentration of approximately 2–4 × 10^8 CFU/ml based on the known concentration of the original frozen stock.
3. Take a firm hold of a non-anesthetized 6–8-week-old BALB/cByJ mouse and pipet 10 μl of the bacterial suspension (approximately 2–4 × 10^6 CFUs) into each nare of the mouse (*see* **Notes 6** and **22**). Monitor the mice over 48 h, at which point optimal colonization has been obtained. The mice should appear healthy and display no symptoms during this time. Any mouse displaying symptoms should be removed from the study.
4. Assess biofilm structure and function according to Subheading 3.4.

3.4 Assessment of Biofilm Phenotype and Function

To ensure an appropriate biofilm phenotype, biofilm formation and function in vitro should be evaluated. This can be performed in various ways (*see* Fig. 2). Biofilms typically contain specific structures of organized chains or clusters of bacteria surrounded by extracellular matrix with pores that allow nutrient penetration into the biofilm and the disposal of waste products. This structural phenotype is most effectively observed by scanning electron microscopy [23] (Fig. 1). An enrichment of bacteria with a lowered metabolic rate [46], together with the matrix-encased structure, makes biofilms highly insensitive to antimicrobial agents and host protective mechanisms [47]. The development of a biofilm phenotype is strongly related to a concomitant and substantial decrease in the expression of genes associated with carbohydrate metabolism and virulence factors and an increase of genes associated with adherence to surfaces, quorum sensing, and competence [43, 48, 49]. Competence and exchange of genetic material can also be evaluated by forming dual-strain biofilms in vitro with strains carrying different antibiotic cassettes or other traceable fitness traits [5]. This section describes methods to evaluate these biofilm features.

3.4.1 Determination of Biomass and Antibiotic Resistance In Vitro

1. Prepare biofilms according to Subheading 3.1.3.
2. Remove the supernatant and add 0.5 ml PBS with or without the appropriate concentration, usually around 500 μg/ml, of gentamicin and incubate for 3 h at 34 °C in 5% CO_2. For determination of the appropriate antibiotic concentration (*see* **Note 23**).
3. Resuspending the biofilm: Scrape the biofilm from the bottom of the well using the tip of a 20–200 μl pipette tip. Float the 24-well plate in a water bath sonicator and sonicate for 2 s to loosen all biofilm cells and disperse aggregates, and further disrupt the biofilm bacteria by pipetting up and down. For details regarding resuspension of the biofilm (*see* **Note 24**).
4. Determining total viable colony forming units (CFUs): Make tenfold serial dilutions (in PBS) for each sample. Plate 100 μl per dilution on blood agar plates and incubate at 37 °C overnight. Count colonies on the plates to determine the CFU per biofilm.

3.4.2 Determination of Biomass In Vivo

1. Colonize mice with pneumococci as presented in Subheading 3.3 above.
2. Euthanize the colonized mice according to your approved animal use protocol (IACUC protocol).
3. Apply ethanol to the fur of the mouse before incision to avoid contamination with bacteria from the fur and environment.
4. Completely remove the fur from the skull and nose using forceps and dissection scissors.
5. Using dissection scissors, cut the maxillary bone (the bone under each eye) on each side. Then, cut through the frontal

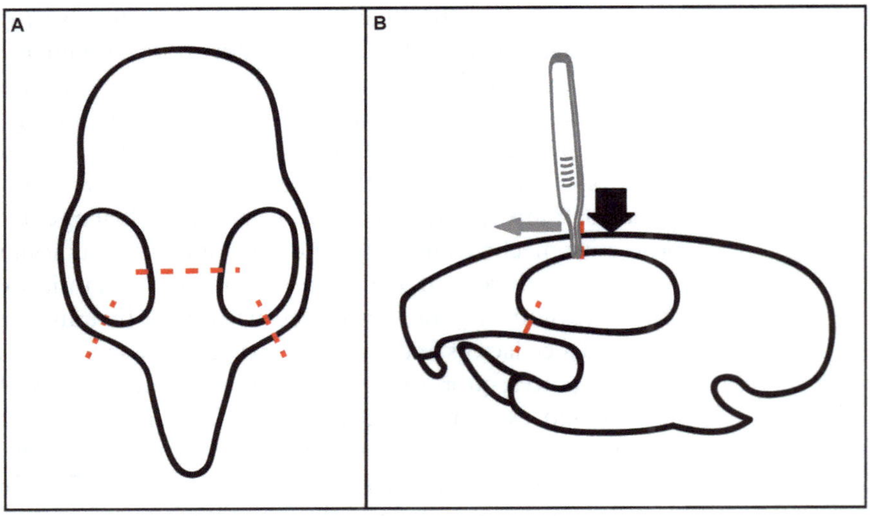

Fig. 3 A cartoon of the mouse skull and how to access the mouse nasal cavity and tissue. (**a**) Top view. After removing the fur from the skull of the mouse, cut the maxillary bone on each side and cut the frontal bone (red dashed lines). (**b**) To access the nasal cavity, hold the skull firmly in place by pressing directly posterior to the frontal bone incision (black arrow; incision indicated by red dashed line) and then insert forceps into the incision and push on the nasal bone (in the direction of the grey arrow)

skull bone between the eyes (just above the nasal bone). *See* Fig. 3a for a diagram of where to cut the bones.

6. Firmly hold the skull in place above the frontal bone incision. Insert forceps into the incision and slowly separate the nasal bone from the frontal bone by pushing the forceps on the nasal bone and away from the frontal bone (*see* Fig. 3b). This separation reveals the nasal concha containing the nasal septum. The morphology of the nasal concha can be observed in Fig. 1b in [50].
7. Using curved tweezers, carefully harvest the tissue attached to the ethmoid bone (medial bone in the concha) to keep the mucosal tissue intact.
8. Place the tissue in a homogenization bag with 1 ml of PBS and homogenize the tissue.
9. Determine total CFUs per tissue by plate counts on blood agar (*see* Subheading 3.4.1 above).

3.4.3 Assessment of Transformation Efficiency in Pneumococcal Biofilms

As mature biofilms express competence genes [43] at a high level, transformation and genetic exchange can occur effectively in biofilms grown on an epithelial surface without addition of the competence stimulating peptide (CSP) [5] (Fig. 4). A study by Wei et al. has shown that transformation efficiency in biofilms on abiotic surfaces increased with external addition of CSP [6]. In the

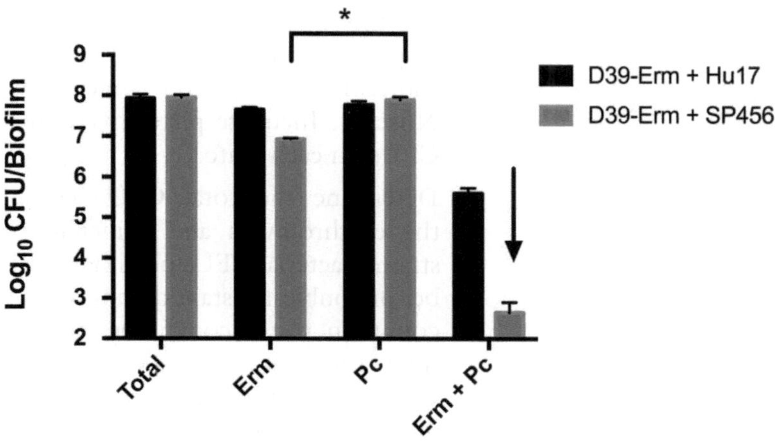

Fig. 4 Transformation of *S. pneumoniae* in biofilms in the absence of externally added competence-stimulating peptide. Two dual biofilms were grown (the erythromycin-resistant D39-Erm strain together with either of the penicillin-resistant Hu17 or SP456 strains). For the combination D39-Erm and Hu17 (black bars), both strains grew equally well as detected by growth on erythromycin (Erm, 0.3 μg/ml) or penicillin G (Pc, 0.5 μg/ml) plates, which resulted in a high transformation efficiency (approximately 0.5%). On the other hand, SP456 significantly outgrew D39-Erm (grey bars) 10:1 (*represents $P < 0.05$), which resulted in an approximately 1000-fold lower transformation efficiency (*see* arrow)

following section, we describe a method to assess transformation efficiency in biofilms.

1. Make sure that each pneumococcal strain used displays measurable antibiotic resistance or has other mutations or traits that can be detected by phenotypic analysis so that strains having taken up and integrated DNA can be detected (*see* **Note 25**). For this example, strain D39 carrying an ErmB erythromycin cassette [51] was grown together with either of two penicillin-resistant strains (SP456 or Hu17) carrying mutations in penicillin binding proteins (SP456; [52]) as well as in MurM and CiaRH (Hu17; [53]).
2. Form biofilms according to Subheading 3.1 for each strain combination. Make sure to add equal amounts of each strain (in this case, one Erm^R and one Pc^R strain). Let the biofilms grow for at least 72 h, as shorter incubation times will result in lower transformation efficiency. For considerations (*see* **Note 26**).
3. Remove supernatant carefully and add 0.5 ml PBS. Resuspend the dual biofilm as indicated in Subheading 3.4.1 above. Before plating the organisms on agar plates, sonicate and vortex the biofilms to disrupt potential aggregates.

4. For this example, plate tenfold serial dilutions of the biofilm suspension on blood agar plates containing 0.3 μg/ml erythromycin or 0.5 μg/ml penicillin G, or both antibiotics (*see* **Note 3**). Incubate plates overnight at 37 °C and enumerate CFUs on each plate.
5. Determine the total CFU (combined bacterial CFUs on the erythromycin and penicillin plates), the CFU of each strain (bacterial CFUs on either antibiotic plate), and the number of double-resistant organisms in the biofilm (bacterial CFU count on plates containing both antibiotics). Calculate the transformation efficiency as the ratio of double-resistant CFUs to the total number of CFUs. A representative experiment is presented in Fig. 4.

3.4.4 Scanning Electron Microscopy of In Vitro and In Vivo Biofilms

1. Form biofilms according to Subheading 3.1. Alternatively, form biofilms in vivo according to Subheading 3.3 (*see* **Note 27**).
2. Fix biofilms grown in vitro or from excised tissue from in vivo colonization in SEM fixation solution for 1 h at room temperature, changing the solution once during the process (after 30 min).
3. Wash fixed samples in SEM wash solution for 15 min at room temperature without shaking. Repeat twice.
4. Dehydrate the samples by adding a series of ethanol solutions (starting at 50% v/v and ending at absolute ethanol in 10% increments) at room temperature for 15 min per concentration prior to critical point drying with carbon dioxide, with absolute ethanol as the intermediate solvent.
5. Mount samples onto stubs and analyze morphology of biofilms and surrounding structures using scanning electron microscopy (*see* **Note 28**).

3.4.5 RNA Isolation and qRT-PCR Analysis of Gene Expression

Since the last iteration of this protocol [19], we have received comments on the difficulty of purifying useful RNA from biofilm preparations. We have therefore improved and changed the RNA isolation protocol to obtain better quality RNA for assessment purposes. This new protocol is presented here.

1. This protocol includes using TRI Reagent, phenol–chloroform–isoamyl alcohol mixture, and chloroform. Remember to work in the hood. Also, dispose of chemicals according to your local chemical waste disposal regulations.
2. For isolation of RNA from in vitro biofilms or dispersed bacterial populations, pellet bacterial cells by centrifugation at 9,000 × *g* for 2 min in a microcentrifuge. Remove and discard supernatant by careful pipetting without disturbing the pellet.

At this point, the pellet can be stored at −80 °C for RNA purification at a later time. Otherwise, continue with the following steps at room temperature.

3. Prepare the cell wall-degrading solution fresh each time.
4. Use a fresh bacterial pellet or thaw the bacterial sample pellet on ice.
5. Resuspend the pellet in 100 μl of the cell wall-degrading solution. Then, mix in 5 μl of 1% SDS and incubate for 5 min at room-temperature.
6. Add 350 μl of TRI Reagent and pass the sample through a 21 G needle five times.
7. Centrifuge at 12,000 × *g* for 2 min at room temperature to remove remaining whole cells and cell debris. Transfer the supernatant containing RNA to a new tube.
8. Add an equal volume of absolute ethanol and mix by pipetting. Transfer to a Zymo-Spin™ IIC Column in a collection tube. Centrifuge at 11,000 × *g* for 1 min. Discard the flow through.
9. Add 400 μl of RNA PreWash Buffer. Centrifuge at 11,000 × *g* for 1 min. Discard the flow through.
10. Add 700 μl of RNA Wash Buffer. Centrifuge at 11,000 × *g* for 2 min.
11. Transfer the column to a new RNase-free microcentrifuge tube.
12. Elute the RNA in 50 μl of RNase-free water. Keep on ice.
13. Add 5 μl of 10× DNase buffer. Then, add 5 μl of DNase I. Incubate at 37 °C for 30 min.
14. Add 50 μl of RNase-free water.
15. Add an equal volume (100 μl) of phenol–chloroform–isoamyl alcohol mixture. Vortex at high speed for 1 min. Centrifuge at max speed for 2 min.
16. Carefully transfer the upper phase to a new RNase-free microcentrifuge tube.
17. Add an equal volume of chloroform. Vortex at high speed for 30 s. Centrifuge at max speed for 2 min.
18. Carefully transfer the upper phase to a new RNase-free microcentrifuge tube.
19. Add 10% volume (10 μl) of 3 M sodium acetate.
20. Add 2.5 times the volume (250 μl) of absolute ethanol. Incubate at −20 °C for at least an hour. Centrifuge at max speed for 15 min.

21. In one movement, pour out the supernatant. While the tube is still inverted, carefully dry the opening of the tube with a tissue and place the still inverted tube on a rack to dry in the hood.
22. Once dry, add 30 μl RNase-free water, allow the RNA pellet to dissolve, and keep on ice or freeze at −80 °C.
23. Verify the RNA purity by measuring the 260/280 nm absorbance ratio in a spectrophotometer and assure that the ratio is above 2 (*see* **Note 9**). DNA contamination can be checked via PCR and compared with genomic DNA as a positive control.
24. Verify the RNA integrity by separating the RNA in a 1% agarose gel, by gel electrophoresis (*see* **Note 29**).
25. For qRT-PCR analysis of the RNA, reverse transcribe the RNA using the Bio-Rad iScript cDNA synthesis kit according to the manufacturer's instructions.
26. qRT-PCR: cDNA amplification is quantified using a Bio-Rad iCycler or similar instrument according to the manufacturer's instructions in the presence of SYBR green supermix and primers for *comD* (competence), *cps2* (capsule production, for biofilms produced using a serotype 2 strain, such as D39), *licD2* (cell wall synthesis), *lytA* (autolysin), and *gyrA* (housekeeping gene). For primer information, *see* **Note 10** and Table 2.

4 Notes

1. The optical density (OD) of the culture can be measured in any regular spectrophotometer with a sterile cuvette (1 cm pathlength). However, we recommend using 16 × 100 mm glass tubes with screw caps together with a Spectronic™ Spectrophotometer that has an adapter for test tubes. This enables quick determination of the OD and also prevents contamination of the culture as the glass tubes do not need to be uncapped for each OD reading.
2. The diluted 80% (v/v) glycerol solution has a lower viscosity that facilitates pipetting as compared with 100% glycerol.
3. To make blood agar plates, mix and dissolve Tryptic Soy Broth powder and Bacto-Agar (according to manufacturer's instructions; BD Biosciences) in water, then autoclave. Cool to approximately 55 °C in a water bath, then add sheep's blood to a final concentration of 5%. Antibiotics can be added at this point if selection plates are needed. Pour approximately 10 ml of blood agar in each sterile Petri dish and let gel at room temperature. Store plates at 4 °C, preferably in sealed plastic bags or boxes to prevent moisture loss.

4. Primary bronchial epithelial cells commercially available from Lonza (NHBE) or ATCC (PCS-300-010) have been used with their recommended media and are useful for validation purposes as well as for producing biofilms on live cells. We have not used Detroit 562 (CLL-138, ATCC) nasopharyngeal carcinoma cells or Calu-3 (HTB-55; ATCC) lung adenocarcinoma cells in our studies, but based on their origin, it is likely that they would also be suitable for pneumococcal biofilm formation.
5. We have adapted the method of preparing CDM from [54] by dividing the ingredients into separate stock solutions (A-E), based on the solubility of the ingredients. Each stock solution contains ingredients enough to prepare 10 liters of CDM and is subsequently divided into 10 aliquots, where each aliquot is added during the process of making 1 liter CDM (Table 1). Preparing material for 10 liters at a time is easier, as some of the amounts are small and hard to weigh out, and is preferable when large volumes of CDM will be used. Here, each of Stocks A–E are prepared for 10 liters in just enough volume (of water, 1 M HCl or 1 M NaOH) to dissolve the ingredients, and then evenly aliquoted into 10 tubes (each to be used for preparation of 1 liter of CDM), and stored at 4 °C. Stock F is also prepared for 10 liters in 200 ml of sterile water and is then stored at −20 °C in 100 × 2-ml aliquots to be thawed and added fresh immediately before use (see below).

   When making one liter of CDM (*see* bottom of Table 1), add the ingredients listed in the left column under the heading "Ingredients for preparation of 1liter of CDM" to approximately 750 ml of distilled water. Add one aliquot each of Stocks A–E, then add the rest of the ingredients listed in the right column. Bring the volume up to 1 liter with distilled water. Filter-sterilize the medium with a 0.45 μm vacuum filter system. Aliquot the medium into 20 × 50-ml conical tubes and store at 4 °C. Bring to room temperature one 50-ml conical tube at a time as needed and add 1 ml of freshly thawed Stock F before use.
6. Pneumococcal colonization has also been successful following nasal inoculation of C57BL/6 inbred mice and CD-1 outbred mice.
7. During SEM preparation, L-lysine and ruthenium red are added to the fixation and wash solutions to retain polysaccharide matrix as described by Hammerschmidt et al. [55].
8. Our protocol is based on the Zymo Research Direct-zol™ RNA MiniPrep Kit protocol. However, we only use the Zymo-Spin™ IIC Column, RNA PreWash Buffer, RNA Wash Buffer, and DNase/RNase-Free Water in our protocol.

9. RNA purity (absorbance ratio 260/280 nm) is most commonly measured using special spectrophotometers, such as the NanoDrop One (Thermo Fisher Scientific) or special inserts to plate readers, but can also be measured in glass cuvettes in any spectrophotometer.
10. As biofilm bacteria and dispersed bacteria differentially regulate genes associated with colonization and virulence, the pneumococcal biofilm and biofilm dispersed phenotypes can be verified by qRT-PCR. We have previously compared the expression of genes using primers listed in Table 2. *comD* (competence) is upregulated in biofilms, but downregulated in dispersed bacteria, while genes associated with virulence, such as *cps2* (capsule production, primers specific for the serotype 2 strain D39), *licD2* (opaque phenotype), and *lytA* (autolysin), are upregulated in dispersed bacteria, but downregulated in the biofilm [14]. The cDNA amplification using these primer pairs was compared with the gene *gyrA* that was stably expressed in all populations in the RNA-seq analysis [43].
11. To distinguish pneumococci from other viridans streptococci, pneumococci are sensitive to optochin and will show a growth inhibition zone around an optochin disc (Sigma) placed on a blood agar plate after overnight incubation.
12. Pneumococci are facultative (aerotolerant) anaerobes and bacterial culture tubes should be capped and incubated without shaking. Avoid exceeding an OD_{600} of 0.6 (late-logarithmic phase corresponding to approximately 3×10^8 CFU/ml) as pneumococci undergo autolysis at higher ODs or prolonged incubation.
13. Preparation of frozen stocks is recommended as compared to liquid cultures seeded from pneumococci grown on blood agar plates. The latter method has a longer and more variable incubation time that is not as reproducible as using frozen aliquots from the same stock. Frozen stock aliquots can be made in different volumes depending on what they are needed for.
14. A temperature of 34 °C is chosen in order to mimic the measured temperature of the nasopharyngeal environment [38]. Also, as compared with 37 °C, we have shown previously that biofilm formation improves at 34 °C for pneumococci as well as for other species residing in the nasopharynx [14, 23].
15. The choice of medium plays an important role in biofilm formation. As shown previously, pneumococci do not form well-structured and functional biofilms in nutrient-rich media, such as THY or Brain Heart Infusion broth [5, 23]. To facilitate the optimal growth of biofilms, we recommend seeding the bacteria as early as possible during the day to enable a first change of the medium later the same day.

Changing medium regularly (at least every 12 h) is of great importance to prevent the pneumococci from undergoing autolysis and will ensure that the biofilm remains stable for up to a week. Although biofilm formation can be detected already after 24 h, pneumococci generally require 48–72 h to form robust biofilms. However, depending on the pneumococcal strain used, growth time and frequency of media change may vary.

16. This is the most critical step of the procedure. During the first 24 h, the biofilms are delicate and must be handled gently when removing and replacing the media. *Do not use a vacuum aspirator.* A 5-ml or 10-ml serological pipette induces less shear force and works better than a 1-ml pipette tip in this regard, both for removing media and for adding fresh media.
17. This wash step is to remove traces of antibiotics from the cell culture medium. Additionally, growing the cells in media without antibiotics for the last 12–24 h will ensure that traces of antibiotics are negligible.
18. For transfer of biofilm bacteria to live cells, avoid pipetting or vortexing the biofilm too vigorously, as the biofilm will re-form faster if aggregates are present. If possible, inspect the biofilm suspension for present aggregates in a microscope prior to inoculation.
19. Change medium carefully as the biofilms are delicate during the process of re-formation (*see* **Notes 15** and **16**). Changing medium frequently is important for the viability of the epithelial cells as the nutrients are rapidly consumed, especially by bacteria passively detaching from the cells and growing freely in the cell culture medium. Using pre-warmed medium (34 °C) is recommended for keeping the temperature constant.
20. Planktonic, broth-grown pneumococci induce epithelial cell death within 12 h of exposure [14]. Based on the downregulation of virulence factors, biofilm bacteria are less toxic to live epithelial cells. The time required to re-form a mature biofilm on live cells varies between species and strains, but usually takes between 24 and 48 h.
21. Frozen stocks are advantageous for these experiments as aliquots have been made and the exact concentration of bacteria in CFU/ml will be known.
22. Preparation for nasal inoculation is most easily done by picking up the mouse by its scruff, then turning your hand over while maintaining a firm hold of the mouse such that the mouse is on its back. Pipet the bacterial suspension slowly into the nares. Mice are inoculated without anesthesia to avoid any aspiration of the inoculum into the lungs, to minimize risk for development of pneumonia.

23. The biomass of a mature biofilm should range between 5×10^7 and 1×10^9 CFU/ml. Reduced antibiotic sensitivity to gentamicin indicates a structured and functional biofilm, which can result from a developed physical barrier to the antibiotic or a slowed metabolism, which renders the antibiotic ineffective. A robust biofilm will tolerate gentamicin exposure well. Generally, less than one $\log_{10}$ decrease in biomass is seen compared with an untreated biofilm. This is in comparison to at least 6 $\log_{10}$ killing of broth-grown bacteria with the same concentration of gentamicin. Importantly, the effective antibiotic concentration may vary between strains. It is necessary to determine each strain's sensitivity to the antibiotic such that the chosen concentration will kill at least 6 $\log_{10}$ of broth-grown bacteria over the same period of time. Gentamicin is used as it penetrates biofilms poorly [56, 57], but penicillin G can also be used at a concentration of approximately 1 μg/ml for pneumococci [23].
24. Use the pointy end of a 20–200 μl pipette tip to completely scrape the bottom of the 24-well plate, using a top-to-bottom and left-to-right pattern. Pipette the suspension up and down vigorously to further disrupt the biofilm bacteria. Avoid introducing bubbles. Sonication will loosen and disperse the biofilm aggregates. However, do not sonicate longer than 2 s as the bacteria may lyse. It is important to disrupt the biofilm bacteria into single cells for accurate viable plate counts. View in the microscope before plating.
25. The example shown includes the transfer of erythromycin and penicillin resistance. Transfer of other antibiotic resistance markers are possible in this assay using appropriate selective media. Additionally, complementation of genes lacking in each mutant can also be detected in this assay and requires the appropriate selection tools to observe. For any transformation experiment, the results of transformation depend on the biofilm-forming ability of each strain in the dual biofilm and optimal transformation efficiency occurs when the total biomass of each strain is similar at the end of the experiment. As pneumococci form bacteriocins, some strain pairs may not be compatible for this assay in vitro. In instances where one strain outcompetes the other in terms of growth rate, an increased inoculum of the strain with reduced growth may improve the end result. Alternatively, growth of the slow-growing strain for 24 h prior to inoculation with the second strain has also been shown to work.
26. Bacterial transfer of DNA has also been detected during colonization of mice in vivo. For this to work, both strains used must colonize the mouse nasopharynx well (at levels of approximately 3×10^6–1×10^7 CFU/tissue) and with approximately

equal numbers. Also, transformation efficacy increases with time so that colonization for 72 h rather than 48 h is recommended.

27. For SEM analyses, grow epithelial cells as described in Subheading 3.1.2, except prepare the fixed epithelial substratum on round coverslips placed into the wells of a 24-well plate to facilitate removal of the biofilms from the wells and preparation for SEM.
28. When imaging the biofilms samples, charging may occur as a result of incomplete dehydration during the sample preparation. To reduce the charging, the samples can be sputter-coated (e.g., coated with chromium or palladium/gold).
29. Separation of RNA by gel electrophoresis should provide two distinct bands representing rRNA as well as a high molecular weight smear of mRNA. A low molecular weight smear indicates degraded RNA that will not work well in the qRT-PCR reaction.

References

1. Koo H, Falsetta ML, Klein MI (2013) The exopolysaccharide matrix: a virulence determinant of cariogenic biofilm. J Dent Res 92:1065–1073
2. Leid JG, Willson CJ, Shirtliff ME, Hassett DJ, Parsek MR, Jeffers AK (2005) The exopolysaccharide alginate protects *Pseudomonas aeruginosa* biofilm bacteria from IFN-gamma-mediated macrophage killing. J Immunol 175:7512–7518
3. Das J, Mokrzan E, Lakhani V, Rosas L, Jurcisek JA, Ray WC, Bakaletz LO (2017) Extracellular DNA and type IV pilus expression regulate the structure and kinetics of biofilm formation by nontypeable *Haemophilus influenzae*. MBio 8. https://doi.org/10.1128/mBio.01466-17
4. Novotny LA, Jurcisek JA, Goodman SD, Bakaletz LO (2016) Monoclonal antibodies against DNA-binding tips of DNABII proteins disrupt biofilms in vitro and induce bacterial clearance in vivo. EBioMedicine 10:33–44
5. Marks LR, Reddinger RM, Hakansson AP (2012) High levels of genetic recombination during nasopharyngeal carriage and biofilm formation in *Streptococcus pneumoniae*. MBio 3:e00200–e00212
6. Wei H, Håvarstein LS (2012) Fratricide is essential for efficient gene transfer between pneumococci in biofilms. Appl Environ Microbiol 78:5897–5905
7. Wolcott RD, Ehrlich GD (2008) Biofilms and chronic infections. JAMA 299:2682–2684
8. Domenech M, García E, Prieto A, Moscoso M (2013) Insight into the composition of the intercellular matrix of *Streptococcus pneumoniae* biofilms. Environ Microbiol 15:502–516
9. Hernandez-Jimenez E, Del Campo R, Toledano V, Vallejo-Cremades MT, Munoz A, Largo C, Arnalich F, Garcia-Rio F, Cubillos-Zapata C, Lopez-Collazo E (2013) Biofilm vs. planktonic bacterial mode of growth: which do human macrophages prefer? Biochem Biophys Res Commun 441:947–952
10. Costerton JW, Stewart PS, Greenberg EP (1999) Bacterial biofilms: a common cause of persistent infections. Science 284:1318–1322
11. Arciola CR, Campoccia D, Montanaro L (2018) Implant infections: adhesion, biofilm formation and immune evasion. Nat Rev Microbiol 16:397–409
12. Weimer KE, Armbruster CE, Juneau RA, Hong W, Pang B, Swords WE (2010) Coinfection with *Haemophilus influenzae* promotes pneumococcal biofilm formation during experimental otitis media and impedes the progression of pneumococcal disease. J Infect Dis 202:1068–1075
13. Blanchette-Cain K, Hinojosa CA, Akula Suresh Babu R, Lizcano A, Gonzalez-Juarbe N, Munoz-Almagro C, Sanchez CJ, Bergman MA, Orihuela CJ (2013) *Streptococcus pneumoniae* biofilm formation is strain dependent, multifactorial, and associated with reduced

invasiveness and immunoreactivity during colonization. MBio 4:e00745–e00713

14. Marks LR, Davidson BA, Knight PR, Hakansson AP (2013) Interkingdom signaling induces *Streptococcus pneumoniae* biofilm dispersion and transition from asymptomatic colonization to disease. MBio 4:e00438–e00413
15. Walsh RL, Camilli A (2011) *Streptococcus pneumoniae* is desiccation tolerant and infectious upon rehydration. MBio 2:e00092–e00011
16. Marks LR, Reddinger RM, Hakansson AP (2014) Biofilm formation enhances fomite survival of *Streptococcus pneumoniae* and *Streptococcus pyogenes*. Infect Immun 82:1141–1146
17. Bloomfield S, Exner M, Flemming HC, Goroncy-Bermes P, Hartemann P, Heeg P, Ilschner C, Krämer I, Merkens W, Oltmanns P, Rotter M, Rutala WA, Sonntag HG, Trautmann M (2015) Lesser-known or hidden reservoirs of infection and implications for adequate prevention strategies: where to look and what to look for. GMS Hyg Infect Control 10:Doc04
18. Dettenkofer M, Block C (2005) Hospital disinfection: efficacy and safety issues. Curr Opin Infect Dis 18:320–325
19. Chao Y, Bergenfelz C, Hakansson AP (2017) In vitro and in vivo biofilm formation by pathogenic streptococci. In: Nordenfelt P, Collin M (eds) Bacterial pathogens: methods and protocols, Methods in molecular biology, vol 1535. Humana Press, New York, pp 285–299
20. Short KR, Diavatopoulos DA (2015) Chapter 15: Nasopharyngeal colonization with *Streptococcus pneumoniae*. In: Orihuela C, Hammerschmidt S, Brown J (eds) Streptococcus pneumoniae: molecular mechanisms of host-pathogen interactions. Elsevier, Academic Press, London
21. Dabernat H, Geslin P, Megraud F, Begue P, Boulesteix J, Dubreuil C, de La Roque F, Trinh A, Scheimberg A (1998) Effects of cefixime or co-amoxiclav treatment on nasopharyngeal carriage of *Streptococcus pneumoniae* and *Haemophilus influenzae* in children with acute otitis media. J Antimicrob Chemother 41:253–258
22. Dagan R, Leibovitz E, Greenberg D, Yagupsky P, Fliss DM, Leiberman A (1998) Dynamics of pneumococcal nasopharyngeal colonization during the first days of antibiotic treatment in pediatric patients. Pediatr Infect Dis J 17:880–885
23. Marks LR, Parameswaran GI, Hakansson AP (2012) Pneumococcal interactions with epithelial cells are crucial for optimal biofilm formation and colonization in vitro and in vivo. Infect Immun 80:2744–2760
24. Ehrlich GD, Veeh R, Wang X, Costerton JW, Hayes JD, Hu FZ, Daigle BJ, Ehrlich MD, Post JC (2002) Mucosal biofilm formation on middle-ear mucosa in the chinchilla model of otitis media. JAMA 287:1710–1715
25. Sanderson AR, Leid JG, Hunsaker D (2006) Bacterial biofilms on the sinus mucosa of human subjects with chronic rhinosinusitis. Laryngoscope 116:1121–1126
26. Hall-Stoodley L, Hu FZ, Gieseke A, Nistico L, Nguyen D, Hayes J, Forbes M, Greenberg DP, Dice B, Burrows A, Wackym PA, Stoodley P, Post JC, Ehrlich GD, Kerschner JE (2006) Direct detection of bacterial biofilms on the middle-ear mucosa of children with chronic otitis media. JAMA 296:202–211
27. Reid SD, Hong W, Dew KE, Winn DR, Pang B, Watt J, Glover DT, Hollingshead SK, Swords WE (2009) Streptococcus pneumoniae forms surface-attached communities in the middle ear of experimentally infected chinchillas. J Infect Dis 199:786–794
28. Charalambous BM, Leung MH (2012) Pneumococcal sepsis and nasopharyngeal carriage. Curr Opin Pulm Med 18:222–227
29. Shak JR, Vidal JE, Klugman KP (2013) Influence of bacterial interactions on pneumococcal colonization of the nasopharynx. Trends Microbiol 21:129–135
30. Gilley RP, Orihuela CJ (2014) Pneumococci in biofilms are non-invasive: implications on nasopharyngeal colonization. Front Cell Infect Microbiol 4:163
31. Chao Y, Marks LR, Pettigrew MM, Hakansson AP (2015) *Streptococcus pneumoniae* biofilm formation and dispersion during colonization and disease. Front Cell Infect Microbiol 4 (194):1–16
32. Allegrucci M, Hu FZ, Shen K, Hayes J, Ehrlich GD, Post JC, Sauer K (2006) Phenotypic characterization of *Streptococcus pneumoniae* biofilm development. J Bacteriol 188:2325–2335
33. Moscoso M, Garcia E, Lopez R (2006) Biofilm formation by *Streptococcus pneumoniae*: role of choline, extracellular DNA, and capsular polysaccharide in microbial accretion. J Bacteriol 188:7785–7795
34. Munoz-Elias EJ, Marcano J, Camilli A (2008) Isolation of *Streptococcus pneumoniae* biofilm mutants and their characterization during nasopharyngeal colonization. Infect Immun 76:5049–5061
35. Sanchez CJ, Shivshankar P, Stol K, Trakhtenbroit S, Sullam PM, Sauer K, Hermans PW, Orihuela CJ (2010) The pneumococcal serine-rich repeat protein is an intra-species bacterial adhesin that promotes

bacterial aggregation in vivo and in biofilms. PLoS Pathog 6:e1001044

36. Yadav MK, Kwon SK, Cho CG, Park SW, Chae SW, Song JJ (2012) Gene expression profile of early in vitro biofilms of *Streptococcus pneumoniae*. Microbiol Immunol 56:621–629
37. Sanchez CJ, Kumar N, Lizcano A, Shivshankar P, Dunning Hotopp JC, Jorgensen JH, Tettelin H, Orihuela CJ (2011) *Streptococcus pneumoniae* in biofilms are unable to cause invasive disease due to altered virulence determinant production. PLoS One 6:e28738
38. Keck T, Leiacker R, Riechelmann H, Rettinger G (2000) Temperature profile in the nasal cavity. Laryngoscope 110:651–654
39. Fux CA, Costerton JW, Stewart PS, Stoodley P (2005) Survival strategies of infectious biofilms. Trends Microbiol 13:34–40
40. Chonmaitree T, Howie VM, Truant AL (1986) Presence of respiratory viruses in middle ear fluids and nasal wash specimens from children with acute otitis media. Pediatrics 77:698–702
41. Diavatopoulos DA, Short KR, Price JT, Wilksch JJ, Brown LE, Briles DE, Strugnell RA, Wijburg OL (2010) Influenza A virus facilitates *Streptococcus pneumoniae* transmission and disease. FASEB J 24(6):1789–1798
42. Pettigrew MM, Gent JF, Pyles RB, Miller AL, Nokso-Koivisto J, Chonmaitree T (2011) Viral-bacterial interactions and risk of acute otitis media complicating upper respiratory tract infection. J Clin Microbiol 49:3750–3755
43. Pettigrew MM, Marks LR, Kong Y, Gent JF, Roche-Hakansson H, Hakansson AP (2014) Dynamic changes in the *Streptococcus pneumoniae* transcriptome during transition from biofilm formation to invasive disease upon influenza A virus infection. Infect Immun 82:4607–4619
44. Briles DE, Novak L, Hotomi M, van Ginkel FW, King J (2005) Nasal colonization with *Streptococcus pneumoniae* includes subpopulations of surface and invasive pneumococci. Infect Immun 73:6945–6951
45. Kadioglu A, Weiser JN, Paton JC, Andrew PW (2008) The role of Streptococcus pneumoniae virulence factors in host respiratory colonization and disease. Nat Rev Microbiol 6:288–301
46. Lewis K (2010) Persister cells. Annu Rev Microbiol 64:357–372
47. Fux CA, Stoodley P, Hall-Stoodley L, Costerton JW (2003) Bacterial biofilms: a diagnostic and therapeutic challenge. Expert Rev Anti-Infect Ther 1:667–683
48. Oggioni MR, Trappetti C, Kadioglu A, Cassone M, Iannelli F, Ricci S, Andrew PW, Pozzi G (2006) Switch from planktonic to sessile life: a major event in pneumococcal pathogenesis. Mol Microbiol 61:1196–1210
49. Vidal JE, Howery KE, Ludewick HP, Nava P, Klugman KP (2013) Quorum-sensing systems LuxS/autoinducer 2 and Com regulate *Streptococcus pneumoniae* biofilms in a bioreactor with living cultures of human respiratory cells. Infect Immun 81:1341–1353
50. Wu HY, Nguyen HH, Russell MW (1997) Nasal lymphoid tissue (NALT) as a mucosal immune inductive site. Scand J Immunol 46:506–513
51. Smith AW, Roche H, Trombe MC, Briles DE, Hakansson A (2002) Characterization of the dihydrolipoamide dehydrogenase from *Streptococcus pneumoniae* and its role in pneumococcal infection. Mol Microbiol 44:431–448
52. Hakenbeck R, Briese T, Chalkley L, Ellerbrok H, Kalliokoski R, Latorre C, Leinonen M, Martin C (1991) Antigenic variation of penicillin-binding proteins from penicillin-resistant clinical strains of *Streptococcus pneumoniae*. J Infect Dis 164:313–319
53. Rieger M, Denapaite D, Bruckner R, Maurer P, Hakenbeck R (2017) Draft genome sequences of two *Streptococcus pneumoniae* serotype 19A sequence Type 226 clinical isolates from Hungary, Hu17 with high-level beta-lactam resistance and Hu15 of a penicillin-sensitive phenotype. Genome Announc 5(20): e00401–e00417
54. van de Rijn I, Kessler RE (1980) Growth characteristics of group A streptococci in a new chemically defined medium. Infect Immun 27:444–448
55. Hammerschmidt S, Wolff S, Hocke A, Rosseau S, Muller E, Rohde M (2005) Illustration of pneumococcal polysaccharide capsule during adherence and invasion of epithelial cells. Infect Immun 73:4653–4667
56. Carmen JC, Nelson JL, Beckstead BL, Runyan CM, Robison RA, Schaalje GB, Pitt WG (2004) Ultrasonic-enhanced gentamicin transport through colony biofilms of *Pseudomonas aeruginosa* and *Escherichia coli*. J Infect Chemother 10:193–199
57. Abdi-Ali A, Mohammadi-Mehr M, Agha Alaei Y (2006) Bactericidal activity of various antibiotics against biofilm-producing *Pseudomonas aeruginosa*. Int J Antimicrob Agents 27:196–200

Chapter 14

In Vivo Mouse Models to Study Pneumococcal Host Interaction and Invasive Pneumococcal Disease

Federico Iovino, Vicky Sender, and Birgitta Henriques-Normark

Abstract

Animal models are fundamental tools to study the biology of physiological processes and disease pathogenesis. To study invasive pneumococcal disease (IPD), many models using mice in particular have been established and developed during recent years. Thanks to the advances of the research in the pneumococcal field, nowadays, there is the possibility to use defined mouse models to study each disease caused by the pneumococcus. In this chapter mouse models for pneumonia, bacteremia, and meningitis are described. Since pneumococci are commensal pathogens found to a high extent in healthy individuals. Hence, we also describe a mouse model for nasopharyngeal colonization.

Key words In vivo, Mouse models, Pneumonia, Meningitis, Invasive pneumococcal disease, Colonization, Coinfection

1 Introduction

Streptococcus pneumoniae (the pneumococcus) is a leading cause of lower respiratory infection and a major contributor to morbidity and mortality worldwide [1]. Mouse models are an essential tool to investigate mechanisms of disease pathogenesis, examine the role of bacterial and host factors, and test novel drugs and vaccine candidates. Recent review articles addressed specific mouse models, like colonization models [2] and models of invasive pneumococcal disease including pneumonia, sepsis and meningitis models [3, 4]. Other authors have investigated mouse genetics and susceptibility to pneumococcal disease [5] as well as the relevance of the genetic background of the bacterial strain for disease development [6–8]. Also the importance of animal models for testing antimicrobials and pneumococcal protein vaccines has been reviewed before [9, 10]. This chapter includes different pneumococcal infection models in mice with a focus on the methodology.

Federico Iovino (ed.), *Streptococcus pneumoniae: Methods and Protocols*, Methods in Molecular Biology, vol. 1968, https://doi.org/10.1007/978-1-4939-9199-0_14, © Springer Science+Business Media, LLC, part of Springer Nature 2019

2 Materials

2.1 Preparation of Bacteria

Before performing the animal experiment, it is important to determine precisely the amount (in CFU) of pneumococci present in the volume dose that will be used to infect every mouse. We recommend plating a sample of the bacterial culture on a blood agar plate that will be used to infect the mice. The bacterial culture can be aliquoted in Eppendorf tubes and stored at −80 °C until the day of the experiment. When defrosted, aliquots are centrifuged at 9600 × *g* for 5 min (room temperature) and then the bacterial pellet is resuspended in 1 ml sterile PBS. The bacterial suspension can then can further diluted in sterile PBS to reach the respective dose/mouse (*see* Subheading 2.2).

2.2 Mice and Facilities

1. Balb/c and C57BL/6 mice are frequently used to study pneumococcal infection. Typically, 6- to 8-week old mice are used.
2. If mice are imported from external locations (e.g., companies), animals are usually housed for 1–2 weeks (resting period) before the start of the experiments. All animal experiments must be approved by the local ethical committee.
3. Biosafety level 2 (BSL2) and animal BSL2 (ABSL2) facilities are used for preparation of inocula and infection/housing of mice, respectively.

2.3 Anesthetizing and Infectious Agents

1. Isoflurane inhalation (~4% v/v) or intraperitoneal (i.p.) injection of 70–100 mg/kg ketamine and 2–10 mg/kg xylazine is used for anesthesia of mice before intranasal or intratracheal (i.tr.) infection. The anesthesia apparatus with chamber for isoflurane is usually provided by the local animal facility.
2. Bacterial strains used are laboratory strains or clinical isolates. All strains are grown to mid-log phase (OD 0.4) in static liquid culture at 37 °C, and aliquots are frozen at −80 °C. Frozen stocks are thawed, centrifuged at 9600 × *g*, and resuspended in phosphate-buffered saline (PBS) before they are diluted to the desired concentration. To prepare 1 L of 1× PBS, start with 800 ml of distilled water and add 8 g of NaCl, 0.2 g of KCl, 1.44 g of Na_2HPO_4, 0.24 g of KH_2PO_4, adjust the pH to 7.4 with HCl, and finally add distilled water to a total volume of 1.
3. The infection dose is confirmed by plating tenfold serial dilutions on blood plates and overnight incubation at 37 °C in 5% CO_2.
4. For coinfection experiments with pneumococci and influenza A virus, a commonly used viral strain is the mouse-adapted influenza A virus PR8/A/34 (H1N1). The virus is passaged in Madine Darby canine kidney (MDCK) cells. Virus stocks are

stored at −80 °C, and virus titers are determined by performing Avicel™ plaque assays on MDCK cells, as described previously [11].

3 Methods

3.1 Pneumonia Model

1. Before infection with pneumococci, mice are anesthetized by inhalation of isoflurane or by i.p. injection of ketamine–xylazine. For inhalation sedation with isoflurane it is important to assess the optimal balance of vaporized isoflurane and oxygen.
2. After the mice are properly anesthetized, each mouse is intranasally infected with pneumococcal suspension [12, 13]. The intranasal administration is performed using a micropipette and by gently releasing the bacterial suspension into the nostrils of the mice (*see* **Note 1**). The volume of the pneumococcal suspension pipetted into the nose is usually between 20 and 50 μl, and the pneumococcal dose is normally within the range of 10^5 and 10^7 CFU per mouse (*see* **Note 2**).
3. In some experiments, to bypass the nasopharynx and ensure that the inoculum reaches directly the lower respiratory tract, intratracheal (i.tr.) infection is required. Before i.tr. infection mice are sedated by i.p. injection with ketamine–xylazine according to their body weight. The intratracheal instillation is performed as described previously [14]. After around 5 min, the mice are observed to confirm that they are fully anesthetized by checking for slower breathing rate, no reaction of extremities when lifted by the neck, and no reaction when the hind limbs are stimulated. To prevent corneal drying and damage, eyes are covered with eye ointment and mice are positioned on a heat pad to maintain the body temperature. For i. tr. infection mice are placed on the intubation platform hanging by its incisors on the wire and gently restrained in place with a piece of ribbon. The mouth is opened gently with the help of a laryngoscope and the blunt-ended forceps are used to gently pull out the tongue. To be able to see the opening of the trachea one gently presses down the laryngoscope and while holding it in place, the blunt ended needle on the MicroSprayer® Aerosolizer containing the inoculum is inserted into the trachea where the inoculum is delivered. The needle is pulled out quickly and the mouse is taken from the platform and placed back onto the heat pad. When the mice are fully recovered from their sedation (takes around 30 min) they are put back into their cages (*see* **Note 3**). After infection, it is important to check that all mice recover properly from the anesthesia and they must be followed up for clinical symptoms by monitoring at least once every 24 hours (*see* **Note 4**).

4. To monitor if the infection in the respiratory tract and the lungs is spreading into the bloodstream, blood samples are collected from the tail vain. Using scissors, a small piece of the tip of the tail (1–2 mm) is cut. Normally a drop of blood immediately comes out upon cutting of the tip of the tail and using a micropipette a blood sample of 5 μl is collected and stored in Eppendorf tubes containing 45 μl sterile PBS (Eppendorf tubes with PBS should be placed on ice) [12, 13]. To prevent clotting of the blood samples, the use of heparin can be considered (*see* **Note 5**).
5. When the humane or experimental endpoint is reached, mice are sacrificed using methods approved by the ethical committee. After sacrifice, the body of the mice are cut and opened through the ventral side using scissors. Organs (mainly lungs) are harvested and collected in Eppendorf tubes which are then placed on ice. For collecting lavage samples from mice, the lungs are maintained within the animal and the trachea is cannulated. The cannula (24G) is fixed with a thread and the lungs are lavaged 2–3 times with PBS alone or PBS + 0.2 mM EDTA. The degree of the pneumococcal infection in the lungs can also be monitored either in vivo or *post mortem* through IVIS imaging [15–17].

3.2 Coinfection Model

1. For coinfection studies mice are initially infected intranasally (i.n.) with a sublethal dose of influenza A virus PR8/A/34 as described above. The infection volume depends on the type of model. For a nasal colonization with the virus a low infection volume is used, whereas for a lower respiratory tract infection a higher infection volume is used to ensure that the inoculum reaches the lower respiratory tract. The infection dose of the inoculum is confirmed by Avicel™ plaque assays on MDCK cells.
2. After virus infection the mice are observed daily for clinical symptoms and their body weight is determined daily. The viral load in the lungs is determined by isolating the lungs from sacrificed mice, homogenizing the tissue, and performing Avicel™ plaque assays on MDCK cells from serial dilution of the homogenized lung tissue.
3. At day 7 after virus infection, which is the time point correlating with the time window when humans are most susceptible to secondary pneumococcal infections [18], the mice are infected i.tr. with the bacterial suspension containing the desired infections dose as described above.

4. After infection the health status of the mice is assessed carefully by observing them closely for clinical symptoms at least once per day (*see* **Note 4**).
5. To monitor if the infection becomes invasive, blood samples are collected from the tail vein at least once a day.
6. When the humane or experimental endpoint is reached, mice are euthanized using methods approved by the ethical committee and samples (mainly lavages and lungs) are harvested and collected in Eppendorf tubes, which are then placed on ice until further processing and/or analyses.

3.3 Bacteremia and (Bacteremia-Derived) Meningitis Model

1. To establish bacteremia, pneumococci are administered intravenously. Bacteremia is the condition preceding the onset of meningitis, which occurs when blood-borne pneumococci penetrate the blood–brain barrier and enter the brain [19]. Here we describe the so-called bacteremia-derived meningitis model which is used to monitor both bacteremia and invasion of the brain by pneumococci, a crucial step in meningitis pathogenesis [16, 17, 19–21].
2. For proper injection into the tail vein, mice should be placed inside restraint devices in which mice are stably locked inside having the tail exiting from the back of the device. In this way, it is possible to handle only the tail, and the mouse can be left awake during this procedure because when placed inside the restraint device the possibility of the mouse to move is impaired. However, mice can also be anesthetized using the anesthesia (isoflurane–oxygen) apparatus and then placed inside the restraint device when the animals are properly anesthetized.
3. It is important to wipe the tail with 70% ethanol prior to the injection. A volume of 100–200 μl is usually used for intravenous infection, and the pneumococcal dose is normally within the range of 10^6 and 10^7 CFU per mouse. If mice have been anesthetized, it is important to verify the proper recovery of the animals from anesthesia.
4. Clinical symptoms must be checked multiple times per day, as stated above (*see* Subheading 3.1).
5. To monitor the degree of bacteremia, blood samples are collected as described above (*see* Subheading 3.1).
6. When the humane endpoints are reached, mice are sacrificed using methods approved by the ethical permits. After sacrifice, to determine the amount of pneumococci that from the blood stream have invaded the brain or have bound to the blood--brain barrier vasculature, perfusion should be performed to remove unattached bacteria in the blood stream. Perfusion is a delicate procedure that is performed by injecting sterile PBS

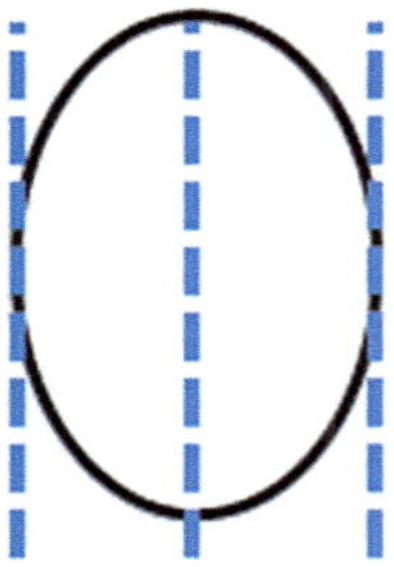

Fig. 1 Schematic representation of how to cut the skull to harvest the brain. The cartoon image shows a schematic view from the top of the mouse skull. The blue dashes show where the skull has to be cut. These three cuts will generate two skull parts that can be lifted using the tweezers in order to expose the brain to collect

in the right ventricle via the vena cava until the blood is completely removed [16, 17]. A volume of 10 ml PBS is recommended to perform optimal perfusion.

7. When perfusion is complete, the head of the mice is cut using scissors and the fur is opened (scissors) to expose the skull. It is important to cut the skull by placing the blade of the scissor between the inner side of the skull (the side facing the brain tissue) and the brain tissue. Three cuts should be performed; one in the middle of the skull, one on the right side, and one on the left side. Afterward, using tweezers, the skull can be gently lifted (*see* **Note 6**) (Fig. 1). This procedure is very delicate since the brain tissue can remain stuck to the skull; therefore, when lifting the skull with the tweezers it is important to check that the brain is detached from the skull. When all the top part of the skull is removed, the whole brain can be collected (*see* **Note 6**) and stored in Eppendorf tubes containing 1 ml sterile PBS. As also described above (*see* Subheading 3.1) the degree of the pneumococcal infection in the brain can also be monitored either in vivo (using white or nude mice, or shaved black-fur mice) or *post mortem* through IVIS imaging [15–17].

3.4 Colonization Model

1. In the pneumococcal colonization model, a light anesthesia by inhalation of isoflurane is sufficient. Mice are held upright and the desired concentration of bacteria in a low volume is administered into the nose using a micropipette by gently releasing the bacterial suspension into the nostrils. The low volume is important to ensure that the inoculum stays in the upper respiratory tract. Similarly, as described for the other infection models, the infection dose is normally within the range of 10^5 and 10^7 CFU per mouse. The mice usually recover immediately from the anesthesia and can then be placed back into their cage.

2. After infection, all mice are checked again for full recovery from the anesthesia and they are then monitored for clinical symptoms multiple times per day, according to the ethical regulations (*see* **Note 4**).
3. When the humane or experimental endpoint is reached, the mice are euthanized using methods approved by the ethical committee. Nasal washes are harvested by rinsing each nostril with 0.5 ml of PBS, and bacterial numbers are determined by plating serial dilutions on blood agar plates. In some cases, lungs and blood are also collected for further analyses.

4 Notes

1. During intranasal administration, even though the mice are asleep, the heart beat can make the animal moving during the procedure. A useful advice is to release the bacterial suspension into the nasal cavities in between the heart beats that usually, during sedation, gives 2–3 s interval without movements. The bacterial suspension does not necessarily have to be administered all in one pipetting but can also be given in multiple steps as long as the mouse inhales the whole volume. In some cases, especially when a higher volume is instilled into the nose, mice are anesthetized with ketamine-xylaxin.
2. The dose can vary depending on the virulence of the pneumococcal strain. Some clinical isolates might have a higher virulence than laboratory strains; therefore, pilot experiments to titrate the infection dose are highly recommended. Also, the scientific question and the desired model (pneumonia, meningitis, or colonization) determine the infection dose.
3. For i.p. injection of ketamine–xylazine the dose can vary depending on the mouse strain and has to be optimized. Too high doses of anesthesia may cause reduced respiration rate which can be fatal. For the intratracheal instillation it is also possible to use a blunt-ended bent needle attached to a 1 ml syringe instead of the MicroSprayer®. If a syringe is used, the volume should not be lower than 40 μl, and it should be loaded leaving an air pocket behind the inoculum to ensure instillation of the total volume. For easier handling it is recommended to prepare the syringe or MicroSprayer® containing the inoculum before the mouse is placed on the intubation platform. Opening the mouth and pulling out the tongue should be done with care to avoid tissue damage. It is important to avoid bubbling of the inoculum. To minimize suffocation and the risk of death the trachea should not be blocked too long. Pull out the needle as soon as possible. The mouse can be held upright for a few seconds to ensure that the inoculum reached the lower

respiratory tract. Care should be taken by applying heat to the mice, especially when using heating lamps. Mice should be observed carefully during the recovery time, and it is important that they do not get too warm or too cold which can also lead to respiratory distress and subsequent death.

4. The mice are monitored for typical clinical symptoms which can occur during pneumococcal disease or other infectious diseases by observing and scoring the animals' general condition (including for example reaction to stimuli and motility), porphyria (red secretion from eyes) and/ or eye inflammation, movement and posture, piloerection, respiration, and the skin of the animals. For virus infection, weight loss is an additional parameter included in assessing the health status of the mice. Scoring of the clinical status must be performed according to Laboratory Animal Science practice and regulations of the institute and the local ethical committee.
5. Heparin can be used when collecting the blood samples, to avoid clotting of the blood. However, it is important to consider that some manufacturers add alcohol in the heparin preparation which can, even if at very low concentration, affect the number of bacteria present in the blood.
6. When cutting the top part of the skull with the scissors, three cuts should be performed in order to be able to easily lift the skull (with tweezers) and expose the brain, as shown in Fig. 1. For this procedure it is more practical to use the tweezers, since using the scissors risks damage to the brain.

References

1. Troeger C, Blacker BF, Khalil IA, Rao PC, Cao S, Zimsen SRM, Albertson S, Stanaway JD, Deshpande A, Farag T, et al (2018) Estimates of the global, regional, and national morbidity, mortality, and aetiologies of lower respiratory infections in 195 countries, 1990-2016: a systematic analysis for the Global Burden of Disease Study 2016. Lancet Infect Dis. 18(11):1191–1210. Published online 2018/09/24 https://doi.org/10.1016/S1473-3099(18)30310-4
2. Malley R, Weiser JN (2008) Animal models of pneumococcal colonization. In: Siber GR, Klugman KP, Mäkelä PH (ed.) Pneumococcal vaccines: the impact of coniugate vaccine. ASM Press, Washington, DC, pp 59–66
3. Briles DE, Hollingshead SK, Jonsdottir I (2008) Animal models of invasive pneumococcal disease. In: Siber GR, Klugman KP, Mäkelä PH (ed.), Pneumococcal vaccines: the impact of conjugate vaccine. ASM Press, Washington, DC, pp 47–58
4. Chiavolini D, Pozzi G, Ricci S (2008) Animal models of Streptococcus pneumoniae disease. Clin Microbiol Rev 21:666–685
5. Kadioglu A, Andrew PW (2005) Susceptibility and resistance to pneumococcal disease in mice. Brief Funct Genomic Proteomic 4(3): 241–247
6. Blue CE, Mitchell TJ (2003) Contribution of a response regulator to the virulence of Streptococcus pneumoniae is strain dependent. Infect Immun 71:4405–4413
7. Kadioglu A, Weiser JN, Paton JC, Andrew PW (2008) The role of Streptococcus pneumoniae virulence factors in host respiratory colonization and disease. Nat Rev Microbiol 6 (4):288–301
8. Sandgren A, Albiger B, Orihuela CJ, Tuomanen E, Normark S, Henriques-Normark B (2005) Virulence in mice of pneumococcal clonal types with known invasive

disease potential in humans. J Infect Dis 192 (5):791–800
9. Nuermberger E (2005) Murine models of pneumococcal pneumonia and their applicability to the study of tissue-directed antimicrobials. Pharmacotherapy 25:134S–139S
10. Steinhoff MC (2007) Animal models for protein pneumococcal vaccine evaluation: a summary. Vaccine 25(13):2465–2470
11. Matrosovich M, Matrosovich T, Garten W, Klenk H-D Virol J 3(1):63
12. Zhang JR, Mostov KE, Lamm ME et al (2000) The polymeric immunoglobulin receptor translocates pneumococci across humannasopharyngeal epithelial cells. Cell. 102:827–37
13. Hentrich K, Löfling J, Pathak A et al (2016) Streptococcus pneumoniae senses a human-like sialic acid profile via the response regulator CiaR. Cell Host Microbe 20:307–317
14. Rayamajhi M, Redente EF, Condon TV et al (2011) Non-surgical intratracheal instillation of mice with analysis of lungs and lung draining lymph nodes by flow cytometry. J Vis Exp 51: e2702
15. Orihuela CJ, Gao G, Francis KP et al (2004) Tissue-specific contributions of pneumococcal virulence factors to pathogenesis. J Infect Dis 190:1661–1669
16. Iovino F, Engelen-Lee JY, Brouwer M et al (2017) pIgR and PECAM-1 bind to pneumococcal adhesins RrgA and PspC mediating bacterial brain invasion. J Exp Med 214:1619–1630
17. Iovino F, Thorsdottir S, Henriques-Normark B (2018) Receptor blockade: a novel approach to protect the brain from pneumococcal invasion. J Infect Dis 218(3):476–484
18. Shrestha S, Foxman B, Weinberger DM et al (2013) Identifying the interaction between influenza and pneumococcal pneumonia using incidence data. Sci Transl Med 5:191ra84
19. Iovino F, Seinen J, Henriques-Normark B et al (2016) How does Streptococcus pneumoniae invade the brain. Trends Microbiol 24:307–315
20. Orihuela CJ, Mahdavi J, Thornton J et al (2009) Laminin receptor initiates bacterial contact with the blood brain barrier in experimental meningitis models. J Clin Invest 119:1638–1646
21. Iovino F, Orihuela CJ, Moorlag HE et al (2013) Interactions between blood-borne Streptococcus pneumoniae and the blood-brain barrier preceding meningitis. PLoS One 8:e68408

Chapter 15

Two-Photon Intravital Imaging of Leukocytes in the Trachea During Pneumococcal Infection

Miguel Palomino-Segura and Santiago F. Gonzalez

Abstract

Two-photon intravital imaging (2P-IVM) of the murine trachea is a powerful technique for real-time imaging of immune cell recruitment and trafficking during airborne pathogen infections. Neutrophils are an important component of the innate immune response that are able to rapidly infiltrate the airway mucosa in response to *Streptococcus pneumoniae* infection. Here we describe a protocol to visualize in vivo neutrophil extravasation and cell dynamics in the tracheal tissue of a *S. pneumoniae*-infected mouse using 2P-IVM. To perform this protocol, we infected and imaged the trachea of a lysozyme M green fluorescent protein (LysM-GFP) mouse, in which neutrophils express GFP. Additionally, we used a custom-designed platform, which allowed the intubation and fixation of the trachea after surgical exposition, and we injected intravenously a fluorescently labeled dextran solution to visualize the blood vessels.

Key words Two-photon intravital microscopy (2P-IVM), Trachea, *Streptococcus pneumoniae*, Neutrophil, Extravasation

1 Introduction

The tracheal epithelium is a mucosal barrier constantly exposed to infectious agents such as *Streptococcus pneumoniae*, which represents a major cause of morbidity and mortality worldwide [1]. Pneumococcal disease is characterized by a primary colonization of the upper airways where the initial encounter between the bacteria and the immune system occurs [2]. After sensing the bacteria, the innate immune system is responsible for the rapid production of cytokines and chemokines in the site of infection, leading to rapid infiltration of highly motile inflammatory cells [3]. Amongst them, neutrophils are the first ones to be recruited. Active migration of neutrophils to sites of infection is fundamentally important to the innate immune system [4]. Indeed,

Electronic supplementary material: The online version of this chapter (https://doi.org/10.1007/978-1-4939-9199-0_15) contains supplementary material, which is available to authorized users.

Federico Iovino (ed.), *Streptococcus pneumoniae: Methods and Protocols*, Methods in Molecular Biology, vol. 1968, https://doi.org/10.1007/978-1-4939-9199-0_15, © Springer Science+Business Media, LLC, part of Springer Nature 2019

neutrophils are able to directly eliminate *S. pneumoniae* [5], which is a critical step to prevent pneumonia caused by the colonizing bacteria [6]. However, deeper knowledge about the mechanisms that drive neutrophil infiltration into the site of infection is still missing due to limitation of traditional microscopy techniques to study cell behavior in vivo.

Two-photon intravital microscopy (2P-IVM) offers unique advantages for in vivo imaging of cells compared with conventional imaging techniques. These include greater tissue penetration, lower photodamage, and the observation of second harmonics generation (SHG) signals [7]. Therefore, this technique has become the preferred tool for in situ observation of immune cell behavior during host immune reactions [8]. 2P-IVM allows for studying important parameters of immune cells, such us blood extravasation and migration, which are related with cellular functions during host defense [9].

Indeed, several surgical models for 2P-IVM of immune-related organs, such as the lymph nodes, bone marrow, and spleen, have been developed over the last two decades [10, 11]. In the case of the airways, imaging remains a challenge due the technical difficulties associated with the ventilation process in these organs [10]. However, different surgical models have been recently described for imaging murine trachea [12–15]. 2P-IVM of murine trachea presents various characteristics that are specially indicated to investigate the cell dynamics of immune cells against infectious agents. For example, the physical location of the trachea, at the initial part of the respiratory tract, makes it one of the first sites for pathogen replication [16] and where the immune response against airborne pathogens is initiated. Moreover, the accessibility and the properties of the trachea, lined by a pseudostratified columnar epithelium, make this organ a suitable location to visualize the initial phase of the immune reaction in the upper airways [17].

In this protocol we explain the 2P time-lapse imaging of neutrophil recruitment and trafficking in the trachea of mice infected with *S. pneumoniae*. We describe the infection of the murine trachea with *S. pneumoniae*, the surgical exposition and intubation of the trachea, and the acquisition of dynamic images where blood vessels, neutrophils and macrophages are visualized.

2 Materials

2.1 S. pneumoniae Growth and Inoculum Preparation

1. Brain–heart infusion (BHI) media + 5% fetal bovine serum (FBS): Suspend 37 g of Bacto™ brain–heart infusion (BD) in 1 L of purified water and mix thoroughly. Heat with frequent agitation and boil for 1 min to completely dissolve the powder. Adjust pH to 7.4. Autoclave at 121 °C for 15 min. Add 500 μL

of FBS (sterile and heat-inactivated) for each 9.5 mL of sterile BHI.

2. 14 mL polypropylene round-bottom tubes (BD).
3. *S. pneumoniae* strain D39 (serotype 2) [18] stock preserved in cryopreservation beads (Technical Service Consultants Ltd).
4. Incubator.
5. Spectrophotometer.
6. Spectrophotometer cuvettes.
7. 1.5 mL Eppendorf tubes.
8. Sterile 1× Dulbecco's phosphate buffered saline modified without calcium chloride and magnesium chloride (PBS) (Sigma).
9. Columbia Sheep Blood Agar (CSBA) plates: Suspend 44 g of the powder (Difco Columbia Blood Agar Base, BD) in 1 L of purified water and mix thoroughly. Heat with frequent agitation and boil for 1 min to completely dissolve the powder. Adjust pH to 7.4. Autoclave at 121 °C for 15 min. Aseptically add 5% sterile defibrinated sheep blood (Thermo Scientific) to the base cooled to 45–50 °C in a water bath and mix well. Aseptically dispense 15 mL to sterile petri plates. Store the plates up to 4 weeks at 2–8 °C, preferably in sealed plastic bags to prevent loss of moisture. Label the medium with the date of preparation and give it a batch number (if necessary).

2.2 Intranasal Infection

1. LysM-GFP [19] mice on a C57BL/6J background.
2. Anesthetic cocktail (20 mg/mL of ketamine + 1 mg/mL of xylazine in sterile PBS): Pipet 5.5 mL of PBS in a sterile 15 mL falcon tube. Add 4 mL of ketamine 50 mg/mL (Labatec Pharma SA). Add 0.5 mL of xylazine 20 mg/mL (Rompun 2%, Bayer) (*see* **Note 1**).
3. 26 G needle 1 mL syringe.
4. Sterile PBS.

2.3 Surgical Procedure for Tracheal 2P-IVM

1. 26 G needle 1 mL syringe.
2. Anesthetic cocktail.
3. Customized surgical board (*see* Fig. 1).
4. Heated plate.
5. Surgical tape.
6. Surgical thread.
7. Electric razor and depilatory cream.
8. Sterile dissecting scissors and forceps.
9. 20 G catheter (Introcan Safety 20 G, Braun).

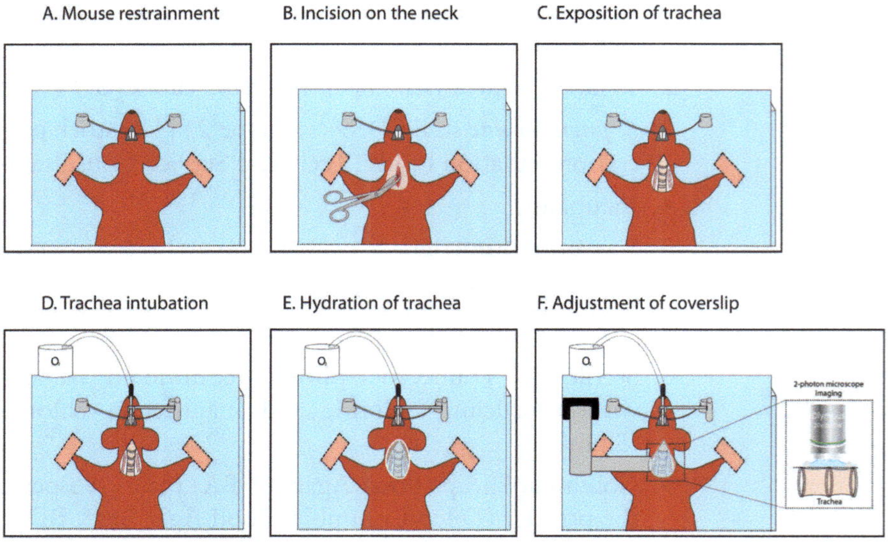

Fig. 1 Steps for 2P-IVM of murine trachea after *S. pneumoniae* infection. Schematic representation of sequential steps for the tracheal surgical model: (**A**) positioning of the anesthetized mouse in the surgical board and hair removal of the neck; (**B**) longitudinal incision in the neck; (**C**) surgical exposition of the trachea; (**D**) intubation with a catheter with artificial ventilation and fixation of the catheter; (**E**) trachea covering with PBS; and (**F**) mounting of the coverslip

10. Oxygen insufflating machine (SomnoSuite® Portable Animal Anesthesia System, Kent Scientific).
11. Petroleum jelly.
12. Sterile PBS.
13. Round coverslip (high tolerance glass coverslip 15 mm round radio, warner instruments).
14. Catheter for anesthesia redosing: Remove a 26 G needle from a syringe using forceps and connect the needle to a piece of PE-20 medical silicon tubing. Then, insert a 26 G needle syringe filled with the anesthetic cocktail on the other side of the tube. Remove any remaining air bubble inside of the tube.
15. 10 mg/mL 70 kDa Rhodamine B isothiocyanate–dextran solution (Sigma).
16. Catheter with 10 mg/mL 70 kDa Rhodamine B isothiocyanate–dextran solution for dosing while 2P-IVM imaging: Remove a 30 G needle from a syringe using forceps and connect the needle to a piece of PE-10 medical silicon tubing. Then, insert a 30 G needle syringe filled with 70 kDa Rhodamine B isothiocyanate–dextran solution on the other side of the tube. Remove any remaining air bubbles inside of the tube.

2.4 In Vivo *Time Lapse and Motility Analysis*

1. TrimScope II Two-photon microscope (LaVision Biotec) equipped with an incubation chamber and temperature controller (The Cube & The Box, Life imaging Services).
2. 25× NA 1.05 water immersion objective (Nikon).
3. Water.
4. Two-photon-data analysis software: Imaris 9.1.0 (Bitplane).
5. 2D scientific graphing software: GraphPad Prism 7 (GraphPad).

3 Methods

LysM-GFP [19] mice on a C57BL/6J background, in which endogenous neutrophils and macrophages express the green fluorescent protein (GFP), were used for 2P-IVM imaging. Mice were maintained in specific pathogen-free conditions at the Institute for Research in Biomedicine (Bellinzona, Switzerland). All animal procedures involving mice were performed in accordance with the Swiss Federal Veterinary Office guidelines and animal protocols were approved by the local veterinarian authorities. In this protocol the *S. pneumoniae* strain D39 (serotype 2) [18] was used for the infection study. Procedures involving the manipulation of the bacteria, the infection of animals or the manipulation of biological samples from infected animals were carried under biosafety cabinet according to biosafety level (BSL) 2 conditions. 2P-IVM procedures with infected animals carried outside of biosafety cabinets needs to be performed in specific facilities with the indicated level of biosafety containment and with the required equipment. Routinely disinfect the biosafety cabinet using UV-light cycles of 30 min and by spreading 70% ethanol solution before and after the infection procedure. Reject solid waste in autoclavable bins and contaminated liquids in specific containers filled with 70% ethanol solution or other any appropriate disinfectant.

3.1 S. pneumoniae *Growth and Inoculum Preparation*

1. Dispense 10 mL of BHI 5% FBS for culture in a 14 mL polypropylene round-bottom tube.
2. Grow *S. pneumoniae* D39 by adding the bacterial stock to the media for culture.
3. Cap the tube and mix briefly.
4. Incubate it at 37 °C in an atmosphere of 5% of CO_2 and grow them statically until mid-exponential phase to an optical density (600 nm) of 0.4–0.5. At this time point the concentration of the culture is approximately 10^8 CFU/mL.
5. Collect 1 mL of the cell culture in a 1.5 mL Eppendorf tube and centrifuge it for 7 min at 4000 × *g* at room temperature.

6. Remove the supernatant, resuspend in 1 mL of sterile PBS, and repeat the centrifugation step.
7. Discard again the supernatant and resuspend the bacterial inoculum in the appropriate volume to reach the desired concentration for infection. In our case, infect mice with a total 10^6 CFU of the bacteria using 10 μL of bacterial inoculum. In order to reach this concentration, the bacteria need to be resuspended in 1 mL of PBS (*see* **Note 2**).
8. Prepare serial dilutions of the inoculum using sterile PBS and plate them in CSBA plates for precise quantification of the bacterial inoculum. Incubate the plates overnight at 37 °C in an atmosphere of 5% CO_2 and count the CFU for the different dilutions (*see* **Note 3**).

3.2 Intranasal Infection

1. Anesthetize mice by injecting intraperitoneally 100 μL of the anesthetic cocktail (20 mg/mL of ketamine + 1 mg/mL xylazine in sterile PBS) per 20 g body weight using a 26 G needle 1 mL syringe.
2. Wait 2–4 min and make sure that mice are fully anesthetized by checking the complete loss of both righting and pedal withdrawal reflex (*see* **Note 4**).
3. Place the anesthetized mice in the biosafety cabinet over its back. Use a pipette to infect with 10 μL of bacterial inoculum containing 10^6 CFU of *S. pneumoniae* D39 by placing the pipette tip close to the mouse nostrils and dispensing the viral inoculum drop by drop. Drops must be inhaled, do not pipette them directly inside the nose cavity (*see* **Note 5**).
4. Repeat the same procedure for another animal using 10 μL for the mock infection.
5. Wait until all the inoculum is inhaled before placing the mouse back in the cage. Check mouse breathing and anesthesia recovery (approximately 60 min after induction).
6. Monitor the welfare of the mice daily by checking the behavior, body condition and appearance. Euthanize infected mice in case animals reach the humane endpoint determined by the veterinarian authority guidelines.

3.3 Surgical Procedure for Tracheal 2P-IVM (See Note 6)

1. 24 h post infection (p.i.) anesthetize mice by injecting intraperitoneally 100 μL of the anesthetic cocktail per 20 g body weight using a 26 G needle 1 mL syringe.
2. Once the animal is deeply anesthetized, maintain the animal on a specific customized surgical board over a heated plate set at 37 °C during the time of the surgery (*see* **Note** 7).
3. Place the animal in a supine position. Fix the forelimbs, the paws, and the tail with surgical tape. Pass a surgical thread

behind the frontal teeth. Next, pull and fix the thread to extend the head of the animal and expose the neck for surgery. Remove the hair from the neck of the mouse using an electric razor and a depilatory cream (Fig. 1A).

4. Perform a longitudinal incision on the neck approximately 1 cm long between the upper chest and the lower point of the mandible (Fig. 1B).
5. Move laterally the skin patches and the salivary glands to visualize the trachea, covered by the muscles. Then, separate in two the tracheal muscles by pulling them with the forceps (Fig. 1C).
6. Connect a 20 G catheter to a tube from an oxygen-insufflating machine to maintain automated ventilation. Set the oxygen-insufflating machine on a breath ratio of 130 beats per minute (b.p.m.) with a tidal volume of 0.2 mL using a 100% oxygen gas supply. Intubate the mouse with the catheter and start artificial ventilation (Fig. 1D) (*see* **Notes** 7 and **8**).
7. Fix the catheter height and orientation using a surgical hook connected to a vertical bar attached to the surgical board. Expose the trachea at the same height of the chin.
8. Surround the trachea with petroleum jelly and cover it with pre-warmed PBS to maintain hydrated the organ during the imaging procedure (Fig. 1E) (*see* **Note 9**).
9. Glue a round coverslip on a metal holder, which will be screwed to the XYZ translator. Adjust the XYZ translator to place the coverslip on top of the surgical preparation (Fig. 1F) (*see* **Note** 7).
10. Place the catheter with the anesthesia cocktail intraperitoneally. Fix the catheter with tape to the surgical board.
11. Insert the catheter with 70 kDa Rhodamine B isothiocyanate–dextran solution intravenously in the tail of the animal and fix it to the surgical board with tape.

3.4 In Vivo Time Lapse and Motility Analysis (See Note 6)

1. Transport the surgical board with the mouse to the microscope incubation chamber preheated at 37–38 °C.
2. Add a drop of water on top of the coverslip and focus on the trachea using a 25×/NA 1.1 water immersion objective (Nikon).
3. Set the scanning frequency to 800 Hz, with 520 × 520 pixels, a field of view of 440 × 440 μm and line average 1. Tune Ti:Sa laser to 830 nm to generate SHG signal from collagen, and the second Ti:Sa laser at 920 nm to excite both GFP and Rhodamine B isothiocyanate. Adjust the power and set up the simultaneous excitation mode (*see* **Notes 10** and **11**).

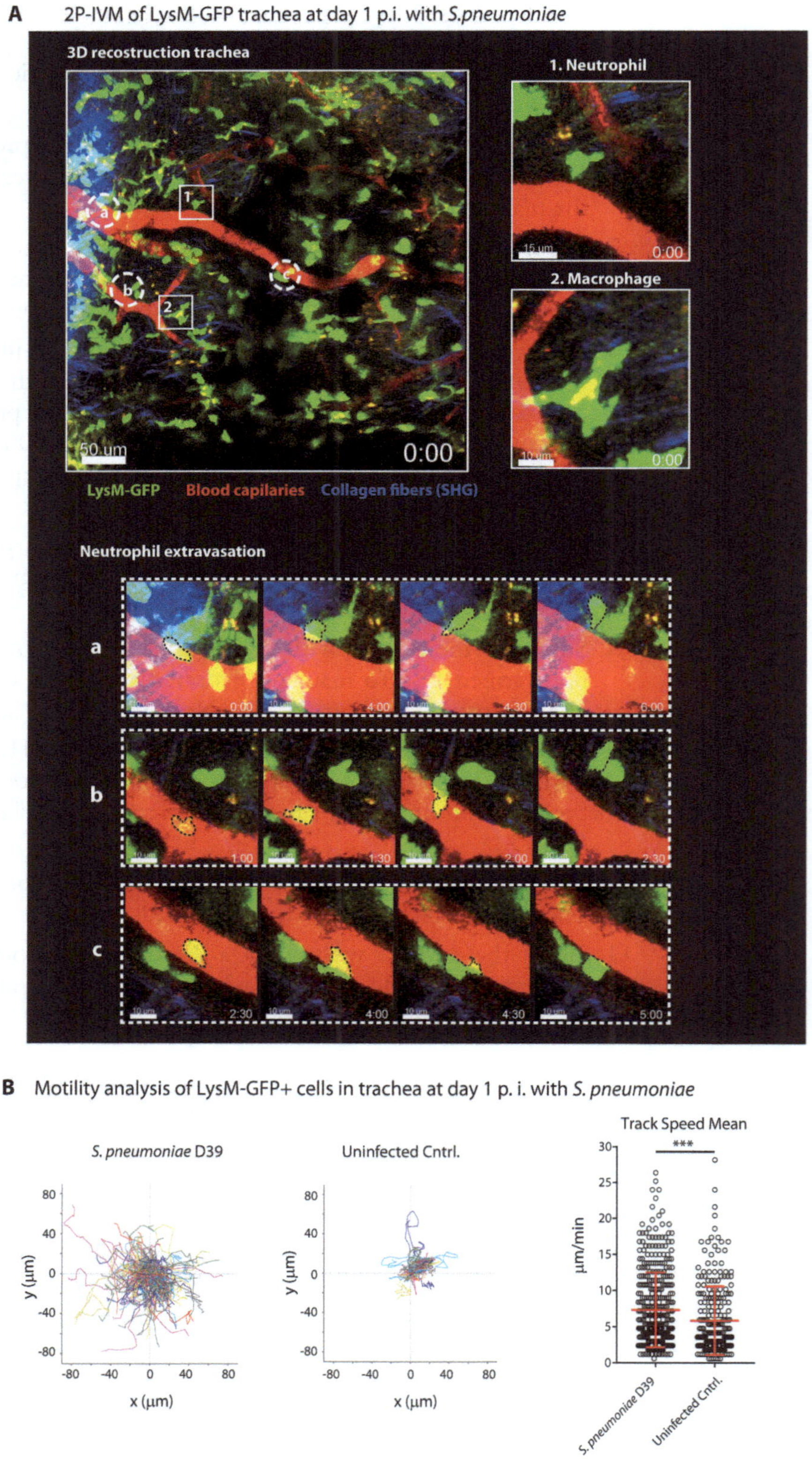

Fig. 2 *In vivo* imaging of neutrophil recruitment and motility analysis in *S. pneumoniae* infected trachea. (**A**) (Upper left panel) Representative 3D projection of a time lapse 2P image sequence showing neutrophils and

4. Define a region in between two tracheal rings with a range 60 μm along the *Z* axis, with a step size of 3 μm (voxel size 0.86 μm × 3 μm). Set up the time between acquisition to 30 s and the number of repetitions to 60 (30 min of total duration) (*see* **Note 12**).
5. Start the imaging process and immediately after inject 30 μL of 70 kDa Rhodamine B isothiocyanate–dextran solution using the catheter placed in the tail vein (*see* **Note 13**).
6. Before running more acquisitions, check vital signs and reinject anesthesia through the catheter if needed (*see* **Note 14**).
7. At the end of the imaging process, euthanize the mouse according to the method determined by the veterinarian authority guidelines.
8. Repeat the same procedure for the mock-infected animal.
9. After image acquisition is completed, transfer the files on a workstation with sufficient computational power. With this experimental setup we will generate to 3D time-lapse images of the murine trachea in which collagen (blue), blood vessels and capillaries (red) and neutrophils and resident macrophages (green) will be visualized (Fig. 2A). Neutrophils and macrophages can be distinguished based on their shape, size and motility (macrophages are larger and immobile) (Fig. 2A1 and 2). Monitor neutrophil recruitment (Fig. 2A abc) and analyze cell motility parameters (Fig. 2B) using any of the available programs and plot the data (*see* **Note 15**).

4 Notes

1. Prepare fresh ketamine–xylazine mixture right before anesthetizing the mice.
2. For different strains of *S. pneumoniae*, perform a preliminary experiment in which different group of mice are infected with different concentrations of bacteria. Then, monitor neutrophil

Fig. 2 (continued) macrophages (both in green), SHG signal from fibrillary collagen (blue) and blood vessels (red) in trachea at day 1 p.i. (Movie 1). (Upper right panels) Magnified areas 1 and 2 show representative images of the two types of GFP-expressing cell populations, the neutrophils (1) and the macrophages (2). (Lower panels) three representative time-lapse 2P image sequences (a, b, and c) showing neutrophil extravasation into the tracheal tissue (Movie 1). (**B**) Graphical representation of tracks with common origin and track speed mean of neutrophils in trachea. Results indicate a major displacement and speed of LysM-GFP+ cells in infected animal compared to uninfected control. Results are given as mean ± SD. Group comparison was assessed using two-tailed Student's t-test parametric tests. Statistical significance was defined as: ***($P < 0.001$)

recruitment in trachea and lungs of infected mice at different time points using flow cytometric analysis or microscopy. In this way, the optimal infectious dose and timing of neutrophils recruitment in trachea after infection can be determined.

3. To ensure *S. pneumoniae* presence in trachea at the moment of imaging, collect the trachea after 2P-IVM and perform serial dilutions of tracheal extracts. Culture them in CSBA plates overnight at 37 °C in an atmosphere of 5% CO_2 and count the CFU for the different dilutions to know the bacterial concentration in the organ [20].
4. Deep anesthesia is necessary for an optimal infection, since not-fully anesthetized mice will swallow or expel the bacterial inoculum, leading to variations in the infection dose.
5. To avoid animal suffocation, dispense small size drops in approximately 20 s intervals.
6. Subheadings 3.3 and 3.4 of the protocol have been adapted from Palomino-Segura et al. [21].
7. Some of the most critical steps to minimize movement during 2P-IVM and to ensure the generation of analyzable 2P-IVM data are: an appropriate mouse anesthesia; a correct mouse intubation; and a surgical exposition of the trachea that allows for an easy access to the organ by the coverslip.
8. The catheter is made by an external plastic part, which protects the tracheal epithelium and an inner iron needle. The needle is an ideal solution to extend and stabilize the trachea and to regulate its exposition. At the same time, artificial ventilation through the catheter will guarantee the breathing of the mouse.
9. Organ dehydration and damage caused during surgery might have an impact on the results when studying the inflammatory response. To prevent this, it is mandatory to hydrate the tissue at all times during surgery, avoid direct contact of the trachea with surgical tools and prevent blood vessels damage.
10. Image acquisition was performed with an upright Two-photon microscope, equipped with two Chameleon Vision Ti:Sa lasers (Coherent Inc.). The photomultipliers (PMT) used for image acquisition were either hybrid detectors or high sensitivity GaAsP. In the setup used in this protocol, SHG signal from collagen was collected in the first channel (emission filter 475/50), GFP emission was collected in channel 2 (emission filter 525/50) and Rhodamine B isothiocyanate was collected in channel 3 (emission filter 650/36).
11. Keep the laser powers as low as possible to minimize photobleaching and phototoxicity.

12. Time in between scans should be adjusted according to the scanning speed of the microscope and purpose of the study. Be aware that a high scanning ratio will require a shorter scanning Z range and will induce phototoxicity.
13. Reinject dextran when necessary to maintain a constant signal in blood vessels. Note that 70 kDa dextran will eventually leak out of the blood vessel; therefore, it is recommended to inject only once image stability is ensured. Dextran with higher size or Qdot® can be alternatively used for the same purpose.
14. Inject 50–25% of the initial dose of ketamine–xylazine mixture every 60–30 min to ensure a strict immobilization of the animal during the whole procedure.
15. For analysis of 2P-IVM data Imaris 9.1.0 (Bitplane) is used. For the representation of the data GraphPad Prism 7 (GraphPad) is used.

Acknowledgments

This work was supported by the Swiss National Foundation (SNF) grants 176124, 145038 (R'equipt) and 148183 (Ambizione), and the European Commission Marie Curie Reintegration Grant 612742.

Authors Contributions. S.F.G. directed the study; S.F.G. and M.P.-S designed and performed experiments, analyzed and interpreted the results, and wrote the manuscript.

References

1. O'Brien KL, Wolfson LJ, Watt JP et al (2009) Burden of disease caused by Streptococcus pneumoniae in children younger than 5 years: global estimates. Lancet 374:893–902
2. Koppe U, Suttorp N, Opitz B (2012) Recognition of Streptococcus pneumoniae by the innate immune system. Cell Microbiol 14:460–466
3. Kadioglu A, Andrew PW (2004) The innate immune response to pneumococcal lung infection: the untold story. Trends Immunol 25:143–149
4. Kobayashi SD, Voyich JM, Burlak C et al (2005) Neutrophils in the innate immune response. Arch Immunol Ther Exp 53 (6):505–517
5. Standish AJ, Weiser JN (2009) Human neutrophils kill Streptococcus pneumoniae via serine proteases. J Immunol 183:2602–2609
6. Matthias KA, Roche AM, Standish AJ et al (2008) Neutrophil-toxin interactions promote antigen delivery and mucosal clearance of Streptococcus pneumoniae. J Immunol 180:6246–6254
7. Zipfel WR, Williams RM, Webb WW (2003) Nonlinear magic: multiphoton microscopy in the biosciences. Nat Biotechnol 21:1369–1377
8. Helmchen F, Denk W (2005) Deep tissue two-photon microscopy. Nat Methods 2:932–940
9. Dzhagalov IL, Melichar HJ, Ross JO, et al (2012) Two-photon imaging of the immune system. Curr Protoc Cytom. Chapter 12: Unit12.26. https://doi.org/10.1002/0471142956.cy1226s60
10. Sumen C, Mempel TR, Mazo IB et al (2004) Intravital microscopy: visualizing immunity in context. Immunity 21:315–329

11. Mempel TR, Henrickson SE, von Andrian UH (2004) T-cell priming by dendriticcells in lymph nodes occurs in three distinct phases. Nature 427:154–159
12. Looney MR, Thornton EE, Sen D et al (2011) Stabilized imaging of immune surveillance in the mouse lung. Nat Methods 8:91–96
13. Thornton EE, Krummel MF, and Looney MR (2012) Live imaging of the lung. Curr Protoc Cytom. Chapter 12:Unit12.28. https://doi.org/10.1002/0471142956.cy1228s60
14. Tabuchi A, Mertens M, Kuppe H et al (2008) Intravital microscopy of the murine pulmonary microcirculation. J Appl Physiol 104:338–346
15. Fiole D, Deman P, Trescos Y et al (2014) Two-photon intravital imaging of lungs during anthrax infection reveals long-lasting macrophage-dendritic cell contacts. Infect Immun 82:864–872
16. Carvalho TC, Peters JI, Williams RO III (2011) Influence of particle size on regional lung deposition–what evidence is there? Int J Pharm 406:1–10
17. Secklehner J, Lo CC, Carlin LM (2017) Intravital microscopy in historic and contemporary immunology. Immunol Cell Biol 95:506–513
18. J a L, Ng W-L, Kazmierczak KM et al (2007) Genome sequence of Avery's virulent serotype 2 strain D39 of Streptococcus pneumoniae and comparison with that of unencapsulated laboratory strain R6. J Bacteriol 189:38–51
19. Faust N, Varas F, Kelly LM et al (2000) Insertion of enhanced green fluorescent protein into the lysozyme gene creates mice with green fluorescent granulocytes and macrophages. Blood 96(2):719–726
20. Iizawa Y, Kitamoto N, Hiroe K et al (1996) Streptococcus pneumoniae in the nasal cavity of mice causes lower respiratory tract infection after airway obstruction. J Med Microbiol 44:490–495
21. Palomino-Segura M, Virgilio T, Morone D et al (2018) Imaging cell interaction in tracheal mucosa during influenza virus infection using two-photon intravital microscopy. J Vis Exp 138:1–12

Chapter 16

IVIS Spectrum CT to Image the Progression of Pneumococcal Infections In Vivo

Adam Sierakowiak, Birgitta Henriques-Normark, and Federico Iovino

Abstract

Imaging through the IVIS Spectrum CT system does not provide the resolution at cellular level like the high-resolution or super-resolution microscopy. Rather, it detects bacterial infections in specific anatomical compartments/organs of the animals. The IVIS Spectrum imaging system is a unique imaging technology that allows for real-time monitoring of disease progression in living animals through the use of either bioluminescent or fluorescent probes.

Key words Real-time, In vivo imaging, IVIS, Bioluminescence, Fluorescence, 3D modeling

1 Introduction

It is important to choose the proper animal model to perform IVIS imaging. Rodents, usually either mice or rats, are used to study invasive pneumococcal disease in vivo. The specific rodent strain used can have a significant impact on the practicality of the imaging. White and nude rodents are preferable, while live imaging using dark rodents can be problematic, although there are solutions to perform good in vivo imaging using rodents with dark fur. Prior to the imaging, anesthetized rodents with dark fur should be shaved with the use of depilatory creams which expose the skin. In this way, the signal obtained is very similar to the one that is obtained using white or nude rodents [1, 2].

To study pneumococcal infections, luciferase-expressing *S. pneumoniae* strains are often used for IVIS in vivo imaging [3–5]. In addition to luciferase, fluorescent dyes that bind to lipids of the bacterial cell wall have been developed recently, and are commercially available. These dyes emit a far-red (near infra-red) fluorescence when they interact with bacteria, including pneumococci (here, we recommend Bacterisense 645 Fluorescent Imaging Agent available from Perkin Elmer) [6]. Prior to the

Federico Iovino (ed.), *Streptococcus pneumoniae: Methods and Protocols*, Methods in Molecular Biology, vol. 1968, https://doi.org/10.1007/978-1-4939-9199-0_16, © Springer Science+Business Media, LLC, part of Springer Nature 2019

imaging of animals, it is highly recommended to perform a pilot imaging study using only the bioluminescent or fluorescent probe. For instance, a plate of luminescent pneumococci or a small sample (using an Eppendorf tube) of a pneumococcal culture mixed with the fluorescent dye (Bacterisense 645, Perkin Elmer) with different concentrations or amount of bacteria can be used and imaged in the IVIS apparatus to assess the detection limit of the bioluminescent/fluorescent signal. The imaging is controlled using the software Living Image (Perkin Elmer).

2 Methods

2.1 Before Image Preparation

1. Animals have to be anesthetized with inhalation of ~4% v/v vaporized isoflurane (*see* **Note 1**). Only when the animals are fully and properly anesthetized imaging can be performed. Mice should be placed inside the imaging chamber so that the anatomical area to be imaged is closest to the top of the animal. For instance, to image major organs, the ventral view is recommended, and the left side is recommended for optimal image of the spleen.
2. It is important to place a black paper sheet on the stage (*see* **Note 2**).
3. If more animals are imaged simultaneously, the use of dividers between animals is recommended (*see* **Note 3**). Mice should be positioned uniformly, and all unnecessary material should be removed from the imaging chamber. Only animals should remain inside the chamber during the imaging process [1, 2].
4. The IVIS system has to be initialized before every imaging. The system usually takes a few minutes to perform the checkup and for the camera to cool down to −90 °C (*see* **Note 4**).

2.2 Imaging of the Animals

1. For bioluminescence detection, the imaging mode, exposure time, binning, and f/stop should be set to the proper level for correct imaging (this can be tested out during the pilot study described previously). If the imaging setup is not known, it is recommended to set it between 30 and 60 s, large binning and f/stop 1. It is important not to image longer than 5 min. If the image is oversaturated, then the exposure time should be reduced. Strong superficial signals can be imaged properly even after a few seconds (5–10 s). The binning parameter helps to discriminate the signal from the noise ratio. It also reduces the spatial resolution, and therefore it has to be properly balanced. The f/stop parameter controls the size of the lens aperture size by regulating the amount of light that the CCD (camera) receives. Also, the f/stop should be properly balanced because a small f/stop value leads to a large lens

aperture size and higher sensitivity, while a high f/stop value leads to a smaller lens aperture size and thus less sensitivity, but better resolution (*see* **Note 5**). A useful and general advice is to use a low exposure time, low binning, and high f/stop if the signal is very bright. In contrast, use a high exposure time, high binning, and low f/stop if the signal is weak [1–5].

2. For fluorescent detection, first the type of fluorescent has to be selected: Epi-illumination is usually used to image superficial areas and is most commonly used. Transillumination is used to image deeper organs/tissues. Then, select the exposure time, binning, and f/stop following the instructions described above for the detection of the bioluminescent signal. Depending on the fluorescent dye, it is then important to select the appropriate excitation/emission wavelength filter. For instance, for Bacterisense 645, excitation is at 635 nm, and emission is at 636 nm [6]. If the optimal filter set is not known, by clicking "Sequence setup" and then "Image Wizard" a user-friendly guide can help through the selection process (Fig. 1).
3. By selecting "Overlay," both luminescent/fluorescent and photographic images will be taken. Also, it is important to select the proper field of view (FOV) to make sure that the animals that have to be imaged are all inside the grid.
4. Rodents with black fur, when properly anesthetized, should be shaved in order to expose the nude skin. Alternatively, postmortem, the body of the animals can be cut and opened in order to image the organ/tissue of interest [3, 4] (Fig. 2).

2.3 3D Tomography (CT Scan)

1. Before using the CT-feature of the IVIS Spectrum CT, one has to make sure to follow local regulations on working with an X-ray energy source. Prior to using the IVIS for CT-scanning, it is important to have a reference scan to reduce the possible error sources and normalize the CT-picture. Start by taking out all things of the stage (e.g., the nosecones and hoses for anesthesia, and the metal plate protecting the transillumination source). Then make sure that the door to the IVIS is properly sealed since one should always strive for minimizing risk for ionizing radiation exposure. Confirm that the IVIS is ready for acquisition and the system has been initialized, as well as that the key on the front of the instrument is inserted and turned to the "ON" position and press the "X-RAY ARMED" button so it turns on (the button is illuminated when it is done correctly). It is always also good to check that the emergency switch (the red knob) is in the ready position (out), and if not turn it clockwise to set it to the ready position. Now the system is ready for the reference picture and if not prompted to take a reference scan, this feature can be found under Acquisition>CT Acquisition>Acquire Reference Images.

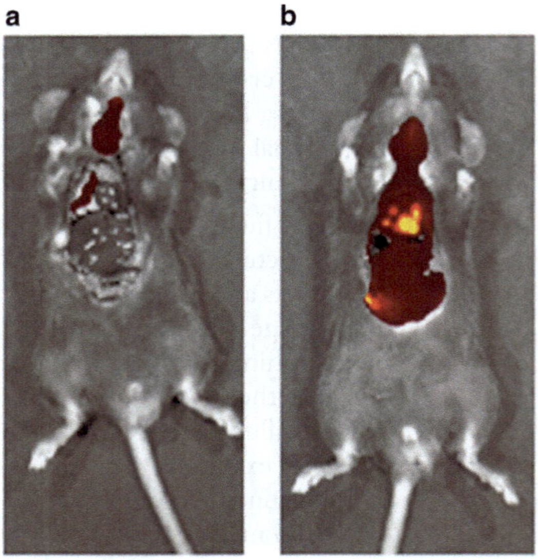

Fig. 1 IVIS imaging of a mouse intranasally infected with pneumococci upon treatment with Bacterisense 645. Two C57BL/6 mice were intranasally infected with pneumococci. Prior to IVIS imaging each mouse was anesthetized and treated intranasally with Bacterisense 645 (Perkin Elmer) (**a**) One C57BL/6 mouse intranasally infected with pneumococci was imaged *post mortem*; the fluorescent signal detected is localized mostly in the nasopharyngeal tract and in one of the lungs, indicating that the bacterial infection remained in the respiratory tract without spreading to the blood stream. (**b**) The other C57BL/6 mouse, intranasally infected with the same dose of the same pneumococci as was used to infect the mouse shown in Fig. 2a, was imaged *post mortem*; in this case the fluorescent signal is not only localized in the lungs, but because the pneumococcal infection spread from the lungs into the blood stream, is also diffused all over the surrounding tissues. The far-red fluorescent signal detected with Bacterisense 645 (Perkin Elmer) results in a scale of color that ranges from dark red (mild infection) to yellow (very serious infection). Fluorescent signals can also be converted to pseudo color scales like the RGB colors generated by the detection of luminescent signals, as described in Subheading 2.5 of the Methods

2. When this is done, the system is now ready for CT-image capture. To start with, the stage for CT-imaging needs to be placed in the middle of the motorized stage and the anesthesia inlet/outlet hoses have to be connected prior to placing the animal. In CT-scanning, to obtain the best result, only one animal at a time can be scanned, thus making this procedure more time-consuming, which should be taken into consideration when planning the experiment. There is also a possibility to scan two mice at the same time, but this is not advised in order to get high quality images.
3. One can obtain CT-images combined with either fluorescence (e.g., near infrared dyes) called FLIT or bioluminescence

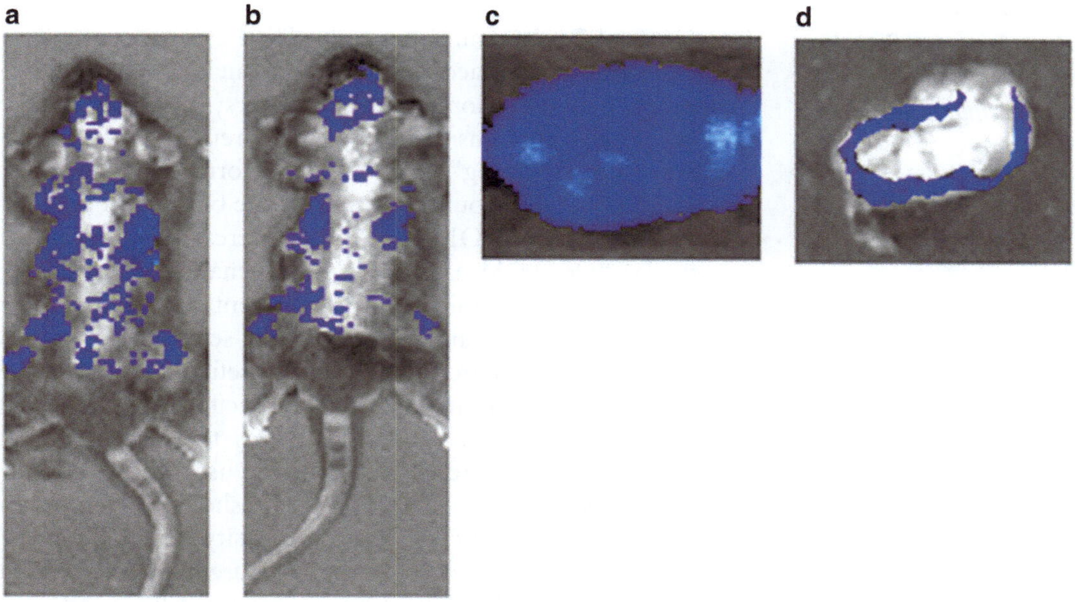

Fig. 2 IVIS imaging of a mouse intravenously infected with luminescent pneumococci. (**a**) A C57BL/6 mouse intravenously infected with luciferase-expressing pneumococci was imaged *post mortem*. Perfusion was not performed, therefore the detected signal is generated from both luminescent pneumococci in the blood stream, and the bacterial infection in the surrounding tissues. (**b**) The same mouse as shown in Fig. (**a**) has been imaged after perfusion, and the luminescent signal has decreased because all pneumococci in the blood have been removed. (**c**) Brain was harvested from the same mouse as imaged in Fig. (**b**). By placing the whole organ in the IVIS chamber, the bacterial signal that is more closely associated to the tissue surface is more easily detected. (**d**) By doing a coronal cut through the brain in order to see the section of the organ, it is possible to monitor the degree of the pneumococcal infection in the brain (the organ is then placed in the IVIS chamber in order to image the organ section); in this case, the pneumococcal infection is mostly localized in the external part of the brain, while the inner brain seems not to be affected by the infection. In all four panels (**a–d**) the luminescent signal detected is blue meaning that, as described in Subheading 2.5 of the Methods, it is generated from a mild pneumococcal infection

(luciferase/luciferin-induced emission) called DLIT. Both acquisition modes can be selected in the Imaging Wizard mode and DLIT (diffuse light tomography) is similar to regular 2D bioluminescence scanning. When doing the FLIT, one has to select what areas the transillumination source should focus on. This feature can be done by selecting pixels in the "Transillumination Setup" during the Imaging wizard as well as the other parameters (similar to the ones described above such as FOV etc.

4. When all settings have been chosen, just click on "X-ray will be produced when energized. Acquire" to start collecting the CT-images in combination with the fluorescence or bioluminescence if chosen.

2.4 Image Processing and Signal Quantification with Living Image Software

1. When the image acquisition is complete, an Image Window and, a Tool Palette will appear. The Tool Palette consents to edit the images postacquisition. The panel "Image Adjust" consents to adjust color settings and scales; the panel "Image Information" contains intensity measurements; the panel "Corrections/Filtering" consents to perform corrections like subtraction of background and modify the binning of the final image; the panel "ROI (Region of Interest) Tool," and in particular "Create Measurement ROI" enable to specifically select and measure luminescent/fluorescent signals of specific regions of interest (that can be manually selected); the panel "Average Bkg (Background)" is very useful to increase the signal specificity by removing the nonspecific signal or signal considered background, and it measures the average signal intensity in a specific area (selected by the user) that is considered as background; the panel "ROI Threshold %" determines the minimum (per cent) peak pixel intensity for a pixel to be included in a ROI. By clicking the Measurement panel/tab a window including all the ROI measurements will appear.
2. Alternatively, it is also possible to analyze 3D ROIs in the 3D-data sets of FLIT or DLIT, acquired with the CT-images. Initially, one has to reconstruct the CT-images and combine them with either the bioluminescent or fluorescent signal and this is easily done by clicking on the tab "DLIT/FLIT 3D reconstruction" and then "Reconstruct." When the entire process is done, one will see a maximum intensity projection map of the CT-images with a combined bioluminescent or fluorescent signal in 3D. Important to know is that one need a separate license for the 3D Multi-Modality tool in order for the reconstruction to be performed. When done, click on ROI tools tab in the tool palette and choose the 3D ROI button to create a 3D ROI. Thereafter click on the 3D ROI transform tool to adjust the 3D ROI to satisfaction. When this is completed, one can get measurements of the bioluminescent/fluorescent signal by choosing "Measure 3D ROIs." For DLIT, choose "3D ROI measurements" Data type: Source Voxels, and choose photons/sec, while for FLIT, choose "3D ROI measurements" Data type: Source Voxels, and choose pmol M^{-1} cm^{-1}.
3. The 3D data can be exported into DICOM-format which can be analyzed with other softwares as well.

2.5 Bioluminescent (and Fluorescent) Signal Quantification by Image J

1. Quantification of bioluminescent signal, generated from luciferase-expressing *S. pneumoniae*, can be performed using the imaging software Image J, as recently described [3, 4].
2. After image acquisition, the bioluminescent signal to measure can be selected using the function "Image-Adjust-Color Threshold" that will automatically generate an RGB Profile

Plot with the intensities of blue/green/red colors. The three colors can be quantified separately, and the intensities of red RGB (red/green/blue, respectively mild/severe/very severe infection) colors are plotted in a histogram which shows on the y axis the total color intensity. Each histogram bar is divided in three parts, one part for each color (red, green, and blue) with the measurement of that particular color in all the points of the area that has been imaged (every point has a YX coordinate on the histogram).

3. Using the imaging software Living Image 4.5, any fluorescent image detected can be converted into RGB colors (during conversion, Living Image 4.5 will show a correspondent scale bar in which it is possible to visualize to what RGB color a specific fluorescent signal corresponds). Quantification of the signal can then be performed as described above in Step 2.

3 Notes

1. To ensure that mice are properly inhaling the vaporized anesthetic, first induce anesthesia of the mice using a chamber (ideally using an anesthesia chamber on a working bench next to the IVIS station) and place the mice inside the IVIS chamber and put their mouth and nose within cones connected to the vaporized isoflurane source (inside the IVIS chamber).
2. The use of a black paper sheet is important to avoid illumination reflections, to keep the stage clean and to minimize infection spreading to other animals/users.
3. Dividers between animals are useful to prevent bright/strong signals to overlap from one animal to its neighbor inside the imaging chamber.
4. During the initialization of the IVIS system, it is possible to monitor the temperature of the camera by clicking on the red bar. When the initialization process is complete, the bar turning green is the message that the camera is at the correct temperature. You can check the current temperature by clicking on the red or green bar.
5. For good quality imaging, normally the f/2 parameter is set at a low value [1] for low intensity (weak) signals, while it is set at higher values (2 or 4) if the signal is particularly bright.

References

1. Poussard A, Patterson M, Taylor K et al (2012) In vivo imaging systems (IVIS) detection of a neuro-invasive encephalitic virus. J Vis Exp 70: e4429
2. Chen H, Thorne SH (2012) Practical methods for molecular in vivo optical imaging. Curr Protoc Cytom 59:12–24

3. Iovino F, Engelen-Lee JY, Brouwer M (2017) pIgR and PECAM-1 bind to pneumococcal RrgA and PspC mediating bacterial invasion of the brain. J Exp Med 214:1619–1630
4. Iovino F, Thorsdottir S, Henriques-Normark B (2018) Receptor blockade: a novel approach to protect the brain from pneumococcal invasion. J Infect Dis 218(3):476–484. https://doi.org/10.1093/infdis/jiy193
5. Orihuela CJ, Gao G, Francis KP (2004) Tissue-specific contributions of pneumococcal virulence factors to pathogenesis. J Infect Dis 190:1661–1669
6. Ravensdale J, Wong Z, O'Brien F (2016) Efficacy of antibacterial peptides against peptide resistant MRSA is restored by permeabilization of bacteria membranes. Front Microbiol 7:1745

Part VI

Public Health, Epidemiology, and Biostatistics

Chapter 17

The Pneumococcus and Its Critical Role in Public Health

Godwin Oligbu, Norman K. Fry, and Shamez N. Ladhani

Abstract

Streptococcus pneumoniae is one of the commonest bacteria that cause morbidity and mortality in children and the elderly. The two extremes of age and individuals with underlying disease are particularly at risk of developing pneumococcal disease. The pneumococcus is responsible for a wide range of infectious diseases, ranging from mild, non-invasive infections such as otitis media and sinusitis, to more severe infections including pneumonia, septicemia, and meningitis. Despite the licensure of highly effective pneumococcal conjugate vaccines, the control of pneumococcal disease is still challenging. Here we describe the critical role of *Streptococcus pneumoniae* in public health.

Key words *Streptococcus pneumoniae*, Invasive pneumococcal disease, Pneumococcal conjugate vaccine, Public health

1 Introduction

Streptococcus pneumoniae (S. pneumoniae, the pneumococcus*)* is an infectious pathogen with significant global burden. It is responsible for over a million deaths worldwide annually. *S. pneumoniae* normally colonizes the nasopharynx but can cause mild localized infections such as sinusitis and otitis media; rarely, the pneumococcus is responsible for occasionally more severe, invasive pneumococcal disease (IPD), which is associated with significant morbidity and mortality. The most common clinical presentations of IPD include bacteremic pneumonia, septicemia, and meningitis. Prior to the introduction of routine pneumococcal conjugate vaccination, an estimated 14.5 million cases of IPD occurred globally in children under 5 years of age, with case fatality rates (CFR) of about 11% [1]. In 2005, WHO estimated that 1.6 million people died of IPD every year; this estimate included up to a million deaths in children under 5 years of age, most of whom lived in developing countries. The magnitude of the burden of pneumococcal disease among elderly people in developing countries is poorly defined [2]. In Europe, in 2015, IPD incidence was highest in infants

Federico Iovino (ed.), *Streptococcus pneumoniae: Methods and Protocols*, Methods in Molecular Biology, vol. 1968,
https://doi.org/10.1007/978-1-4939-9199-0_17,

(12.9 cases per 100,000 population) and the elderly (16.1 cases per 100,000 population) [3].

IPD generally is associated with significant case fatality and, of those who survive, high proportions suffer long-term complications, especially those presenting with meningitis. In a global review, about 25% (IQR 16%, 35%) of pneumococcal meningitis cases developed major neurological sequelae [4]. Similar findings were reported in a systematic review of literature from African countries, where about one-quarter of children surviving pneumococcal meningitis had serious neurological sequelae at the time of hospital discharge [5]. Almost 100 different pneumococcal serotypes have been identified. A pneumococcal conjugate vaccine against the seven most prevalent serotypes (PCV7) causing IPD in young children was first introduced into the childhood immunization programme in the USA in 2000. Other countries subsequently adopted the vaccine at different times. PCV7 has been highly effective in preventing IPD caused by the vaccine serotypes across all age groups through direct and indirect (herd) protection. PCV7 has subsequently been replaced with 10-valent (PCV10) and 13-valent (PCV13) vaccines. With all the PCVs, the reduction in PCV-type IPD has been offset by an increase in IPD caused by non-vaccine serotypes (NVT). In this chapter, we describe the critical role of *Streptococcus pneumoniae* in public health and the global burden of IPD.

2 Material and Methods

2.1 Search Strategy

A search strategy was undertaken to define the global burden of invasive pneumococcal disease and the impact of vaccination in countries with established PCV immunization programs. We searched MEDLINE, EMBASE, and the Cochrane library from 1st January 2000 to 30th April 2016, as well as the ISI web of knowledge, to identify relevant articles and conference proceedings. The medical subject headings (MeSH) terms used included "invasive pneumococcal disease," "Streptococcus pneumoniae," "pneumococcus," "pneumococcal infection," "epidemiology," "burden," and "surveillance." We included studies published in English language. In addition, we screened reference lists of selected papers to retrieve relevant studies.

Studies were eligible for inclusion if they reported population estimates of disease burden and from observational studies and surveillance databases. The title and abstracts of all identified publications were screened, and full articles of included publications were retrieved and reviewed for eligibility. Eligible studies were then assessed according to the Reporting Items for Systematic Reviews and Meta-analyses (PRISMA) statement for the conduct and reporting of systematic reviews.

2.2 Case Definition

A case of IPD was defined as identification of *S. pneumoniae* (by culture, PCR, or antigen testing) from a normally sterile site (e.g., blood, cerebrospinal fluid, or, less commonly, joint, pleural, or pericardial fluid). Because pneumococci frequently colonize the upper respiratory tract in the absence of disease, the clinical significance of recovering the organism from non-sterile body sites (e.g., expectorated sputum, conjunctiva) is less certain. Detection of pneumococcal capsular antigen in urine may be useful for the diagnosis of pneumococcal pneumonia in older children and adults, but may yield false positive results in infants and young children because of high pneumococcal carriage rates in this age group.

2.3 Serotyping

A variety of laboratory methods are used to serotype strains, such as Quellung, Pneumotest®, slide agglutination, latex agglutination, coagglutination, multiplex PCR, and gel diffusion [6]. More recently, whole-genome sequence analysis has been used to predict serotype and provide detailed genetic information of infecting strains [7].

2.4 Case Reporting

Different countries have regulations and laws governing the reporting of IPD and other diseases and conditions of public health importance. Most countries currently require IPD to be reported to designated regional, state or public health authorities, regardless of the age of the patient or presence of drug resistance. Some countries require reporting in limited populations, such as children <5 years of age. Healthcare providers identify cases of IPD through microbiology laboratories, death certificates, and hospital discharge.

3 Findings

3.1 The History of Pneumococcus

The pneumococcus was first isolated by the US Army physician George Sternberg and the French chemist Louis Pasteur in 1886 independently, following its role as a major cause of pneumonia [8, 9]. In 1920, due to its characteristic appearance on Gram stain, it was renamed *Diplococcus pneumoniae* [10], which was changed to *Streptococci pneumoniae* in 1974, since it had similar features to other bacteria in the streptococcus group.

S. pneumoniae has played a critical role in human disease. Its capsular polysaccharide is known to be pivotal to its virulence. This was established as far back as 1931 by Avery and colleagues using an enzyme obtained from a soil bacillus that removed the serotype 3 capsular polysaccharide [11]. These findings and work by other scientists opened the door for a number of studies in the 1930s and 1940s on vaccines aimed at preventing pneumococcal disease. In 1937, for example, Felton's capsular material was successfully used in a program of mass vaccination to abort an outbreak of pneumonia at a state hospital [12].

In addition, the discovery of the antibacterial properties of the fungus-derived substance that came to be called penicillin by Fleming in 1929 completely changed the approach to treatment of pneumococcal infections [13]. This led to great successes in the treatment of a variety of staphylococcal and streptococcal (including pneumococcal) infections, especially those resistant to sulfonamides [14].

However, penicillin-resistant pneumococcal strains emerged in the 1960s and 1970s. The mechanism by which resistance to penicillin arises in pneumococci involves decreased binding of the drug to penicillin binding proteins (PBPs), which are also known as transmembrane carboxypeptidases-enzymes involved in cell wall synthesis [15]. This virulent ability and transforming principle of pneumococcus was first described in 1916 by Stryker [16].

Later, Hotchkiss [17] showed that, in addition to the genes encoding capsule production, those sequences encoding resistance to penicillin could be transferred to a previously penicillin-sensitive pneumococcus by DNA isolated from a penicillin-resistant pneumococcus. The increasing incidence of penicillin-resistant pneumococci continues globally. New antibiotics, as well as different preventive and therapeutic strategies, therefore, needed to be developed to combat this trend.

3.2 The Pneumococcus and Serotypes

S. pneumoniae is a Gram-positive, encapsulated diplococcus. The polysaccharide capsule of this bacterium is an essential virulence factor for invasive disease. The unique polysaccharide capsule is used to distinguish between the different pneumococcal strains serologically. Almost 100 different pneumococcal serotypes have been identified, and most serotypes can cause invasive and non-invasive disease. Although there are significant geographical variations, with different serotypes dominating in different regions, common serotypes are consistently identified throughout the world. These variations are the results of age, time and possible environmental influence [18]. In children, prior to routine pneumococcal conjugate vaccination, the seven most common serotypes were responsible for 60–80% of all IPD [19].

S. pneumoniae resides asymptomatically in the nasopharynx of healthy carriers without causing any symptoms. The organism is transmitted by direct contact with respiratory secretions from patients and healthy carriers. Transient nasopharyngeal colonization, not disease, is the normal outcome of exposure to pneumococci. The highest carriage rates are in young children, with reported rates of 30–50% in industrialized countries [20]. Factors associated with higher carriage rates include age <2 years, nursery attendance and out-of-home childcare, crowding, winter season and parental smoking [21]. Occasionally, *S. pneumoniae* may invade locally to cause non-invasive mucosal infections such as sinusitis, otitis media, and non-bacteremic pneumonia. In susceptible individuals, particularly the immunocompromised, older adults and young children, *S. pneumoniae* infection can lead to invasive disease, including septicemia, bacteremic pneumonia, and meningitis, as well as other less common secondary localized infections such as septic arthritis, osteomyelitis, endocarditis, and periorbital cellulitis [22].

The pneumococcus is the commonest cause of community-acquired pneumonia in adults, although the actual proportion proven to be caused by this organism varies depending on the region and population under study. In developing countries, non-bacteremic pneumonia causes the majority of pneumococcal deaths in children. It is also the commonest cause of bacterial meningitis in adults and second most common cause in young children after meningococcal meningitis.

Streptococcus pneumoniae is an uncommon but recognized cause of puerperal sepsis, with significant maternal and infant morbidity and mortality. Both early and late onset disease have been reported [23]. Unlike group B streptococci, however, *S. pneumoniae* rarely colonizes the female genital tract but has a very high infant invasion to maternal colonization ratio [24].

Recent acquisition of the pneumococcus is associated with IPD, although, not all pneumococcal types are equally invasive; the composition and quantity of capsular polysaccharide has a major role in virulence and invasive potential. Thus, while certain serotypes are infrequently isolated from the nasopharynx, they contribute disproportionately to IPD. In large studies, serotypes 1, 2, 4, 5, 7F, 8, 9,12F, 14, 16, 18C, and 19A were found to be more invasive compared to serotypes 3, 6A, 6B, 11A, 15B/C, 19, and 23F, which were generally less invasive [25–30].

Population-based studies have identified significant associations between specific pneumococcal serotypes and disease severity (e.g., death) among patients with septicemia [31] pneumonia [32], and meningitis [33]. A recent meta-analysis evaluated serotype-specific outcomes and found that serotypes 1, 7F, and 8 were associated with lower odds of death, whereas serotypes 3, 6A, 6B, 9N, and 19F were associated with a higher risk of death [32].

In the USA, prior to the widespread use of PCVs, the case fatality rate for pneumococcal pneumonia was 5%, increasing to 20% for septicemia and 30% for meningitis [34]. A major risk factor for death with IPD is the presence of underlying comorbidities. In a recent observational study in the UK, clinical presentation with meningitis and the presence of comorbidity were independent risk factors for death in children with IPD [35]. IPD-related CFR was 8.5% in children with comorbidities compared with 3.5% in those without [36].

3.3 Risk Factors for Invasive Pneumococcal Disease

Certain groups of people are at higher risk of IPD. In the USA prior to the introduction of PCV7, African American, Alaska Natives, and some American Indian populations had increased risk of IPD compared with white people. The extent to which increased risks are attributable to factors other than race and ethnicity are not clear. The increased risks of race persist despite controlling for income [37]. In one study, IPD was more common in blacks than in whites [38].

In addition, a number of case control studies have also demonstrated a strong associations of IPDs with the presence of underlying disease, environmental factors, larger family size, and with attendance at out-of-home childcare in preceding 3 months, suggesting that factors other than ethnicity also contribute to a higher risk [39]. Children with sickle cell disease (SCD) or with human immunodeficiency virus (HIV) infections, especially ≤2 year-olds, have markedly higher incidence of IPD, as do those with asplenia, nephrotic syndrome, immunodeficiency other than HIV, immunosuppressive therapy and conditions associated with cerebrospinal fluid leak. Children with a cochlear implant, in particular those who received an implant with positioner, also have an increased risk of pneumococcal meningitis [40].

In a study assessing the risk of IPD in HIV infected children, a 9- to 43-fold increased relative risk of IPD was observed [41]. Even with the routine use of highly active retroviral therapy (HAART), the incidence of IPD was only reduced by 50% in HIV-infected children compared to age matched, HIV uninfected children [42]. A much higher risk has also been reported in a population study of children with SCD in the UK, who had a four-fold increase risk of IPD and were five times more likely to die from IPD, even in the era of national pneumococcal conjugate vaccine programs and routine childhood penicillin prophylaxis recommendations [43].

4 Conclusion

The introduction of conjugate vaccines into national childhood immunization programs led to large and sustained decline in infections caused by *Haemophilus influenzae* type b (Hib) and group C meningococcal (MenC) disease. *Streptococcus pneumoniae* remains a major cause of morbidity and mortality worldwide, especially at the extremes of age and in individuals with underlying comorbidity. The control of pneumococcal disease through vaccination, however, has been more challenging. The large number of pneumococcal serotypes that can cause serious disease, their varied virulent capability, and increasing antibiotic resistance remain the main challenge in developing strategies to control this pathogen of global importance.

References

1. O'Brien KL, Wolfson LJ, Watt JP, Henkle E, Deloria-Knoll M, McCall N et al (2009) Burden of disease caused by Streptococcus pneumoniae in children younger than 5 years: global estimates. Lancet 374(9693):893–902
2. World Health Organization (2007) Pneumococcal conjugate vaccine for childhood immunization - WHO position paper. Wkly Epidemiol Rec 82(12):93–104
3. European Centre for Disease Prevention and Control (2017) Invasive pneumococcal disease. Stockholm. https://ecdc.europa.eu/en/publications-data/invasive-pneumococcal-disease-annual-epidemiological-report-2017. Accessed 12 May 2018
4. Edmond K, Clark A, Korczak VS et al (2010) Global and regional risk of disabling sequelae from bacterial meningitis: a systematic review and meta-analysis. Lancet Infect Dis 10:317–328
5. Ramakrishnan M, Ulland AJ, Steinhardt LC, Moïsi JC, Were F et al (2009) Sequelae due to bacterial meningitis among African children: a systematic literature review. BMC Med 7(1):47
6. Jauneikaite E, Tocheva AS, Jefferies JM, Gladstone RA, Faust SN, Christodoulides M et al (2015) Current methods for capsular typing of Streptococcus pneumoniae. J Microbiol Methods 113:41–49. https://doi.org/10.1016/j.mimet.2015.03.006. Epub 2015 Mar 25
7. Kapatai G, Sheppard CL, Al-Shahib A, Litt DJ, Underwood AP, Harrison TG et al (2016) Whole genome sequencing of Streptococcus pneumoniae: development, evaluation and verification of targets for serogroup and serotype prediction using an automated pipeline. PeerJ 4:e2477. https://doi.org/10.7717/peerj.2477. eCollection 2016
8. Sternberg GM (1881) A fatal form of septicaemia in the rabbit produced by the subcutaneous injection of human saliva: an experimental research. John Murphy Co., Baltimore
9. Pasteur L (1881) Sur une maladie nouvelle, provoqué par la salive dún enfant mort de la rage. C R Acad Sci 92:159
10. Winslow CE, Broadhurst J, Buchanan RE, Krumwiede C, Rogers LA, Smith GH (1920) The families and genera of the bacteria: final report of the committee of the society of American bacteriologists on characterization and classification of bacterial types. J Bacteriol 5 (3):191–229
11. Avery OT, Dubos R (1931) The protective action of a specific enzyme against type III pneumococcus infections in mice. J Exp Med 54:73–89
12. Smillie WG, Warnock GH, White HJ (1938) A study of a type I pneumococcus epidemic at the state hospital at Worcester, Mass. Am J Public Health Nations Health 28(3):293–302
13. Fleming A (1929) On the antibacterial action of cultures of a penicillin, with special reference to their use in isolation of B. influenzae. Br J Exp Pathol 10(3):226–236
14. Keefer CS, Blake FG, Marshall EK Jr, Lockwood JS, Wood BW Jr (1943) Penicillin in the treatment of infections: a report of 500 cases. JAMA 122:1217–1224
15. Jacobs MR, Koornhof HJ, Robins-Browne RM et al (1978) Emergence of multiply resistant pneumococci. N Engl J Med 299:735–740
16. Stryker LM (1916) Variations in the pneumococcus induced by growth in immune serum. J Exp Med 24:49–68
17. Hotchkiss RD (1951) Transfer of penicillin resistance in pneumococci by the desoxyribonucleate derived from resistant cultures. Cold Spring Harb Symp Quant Biol 16:457–461
18. Hausdorff WP, Bryant J, Paradiso PR, Siber GR (2000) Which pneumococcal serogroups cause the most invasive disease: implications for conjugate vaccine formulation and use, part I. Clin Infect Dis 30(1):100–121
19. Robbins JB, Austrian R, Lee CJ, Rastogi SC, Schiffman G, Henrichsen J et al (1983) Considerations for formulating the second-generation pneumococcal capsular polysaccharide vaccine with emphasis on the cross-reactive types within groups. J Infect Dis 148 (6):1136–1159
20. Van Hoek AJ, Sheppard CL, Andrews NJ, Waight PA, Slack MPE, Harrison TG et al (2014) Pneumococcal carriage in children and adults two years after introduction of the thirteen valent pneumococcal conjugate vaccine in England. Vaccine 32(34):4349–4355
21. Lexau CA, Lynfield R, Danila R, Pilishvili T, Facklam R, Farley MM et al (2005) Changing epidemiology of invasive pneumococcal disease among older adults in the era of pediatric pneumococcal conjugate vaccine. JAMA 294 (16):2043–2051
22. Advisory Committee on Immunization Practices (2000) Preventing pneumococcal disease

among infants and young children. Recommendations of the advisory committee on immunization practices (ACIP). MMWR Recomm Rep 49(RR-9):1–35

23. Deutscher M, Lewis M, Zell ER, Taylor TH Jr, Van Beneden C et al (2011) Incidence and severity of invasive streptococcus pneumoniae, group A streptococcus, and group B streptococcus infections among pregnant and postpartum women. Clin Infect Dis 53(2):114–123
24. Ladhani SN, Andrews NJ, Waight P, Borrow R, Slack MP, Miller E (2012) Impact of the 7-valent pneumococcal conjugate vaccine on invasive pneumococcal disease in infants younger than 90 days in England and Wales. Clin Infect Dis 56(5):633–640
25. Kronenberg A, Zucs P, Droz S, Muhlemann K (2006) Distribution and invasiveness of Streptococcus pneumoniae serotypes in Switzerland, a country with low antibiotic selection pressure, from 2001 to 2004. J Clin Microbiol 44 (6):2032–2038
26. Sleeman KL, Griffiths D, Shackley F, Diggle L, Gupta S, Maiden MC et al (2006) Capsular serotype-specific attack rates and duration of carriage of Streptococcus pneumoniae in a population of children. J Infect Dis 194 (5):682–688
27. Brueggemann AB, Griffiths DT, Meats E, Peto T, Crook DW et al (2003) Clonal relationships between invasive and carriage Streptococcus pneumoniae and serotype- and clone-specific differences in invasive disease potential. J Infect Dis 187(9):1424–1432
28. Sá-Leão R, Pinto F, Aguiar S, Nunes S, Carriço JA, Frazão N et al (2011) Analysis of invasiveness of pneumococcal serotypes and clones circulating in Portugal before widespread use of conjugate vaccines reveals heterogeneous behavior of clones expressing the same serotype. J Clin Microbiol 49(4):1369–1375
29. Rivera-Olivero IA, del Nogal B, Sisco MC, Bogaert D, Hermans PW et al (2011) Carriage and invasive isolates of Streptococcus pneumoniae in Caracas, Venezuela: the relative invasiveness of serotypes and vaccine coverage. Eur J Clin Microbiol Infect Dis 30 (12):1489–1495
30. Yildirim I, Hanage WP, Lipsitch M, Shea KM, Stevenson A, Finkelstein J et al (2010) Serotype specific invasive capacity and persistent reduction in invasive pneumococcal disease. Vaccine 29:283–288
31. Harboe ZB, Thomsen RW, Riis A, Valentiner-Branth P, Christensen JJ, Lambertsen L et al (2009) Pneumococcal serotypes and mortality following invasive pneumococcal disease: a population-based cohort study. PLoS Med 6 (5):e1000081–e1000081
32. Weinberger DM, Harboe ZB, Sanders EAM, Ndiritu M, Klugman KP, Rückinger S et al (2010) Association of serotype with risk of death due to pneumococcal pneumonia: a meta-analysis. Clin Infect Dis 51(6):692–699
33. Oligbu G, Djennad A, Collins S, Sheppard NK, Fry NK, Borrow R et al (2018) Impact of pneumococcal conjugate vaccines on pneumococcal meningitis in England and Wales, 2000–2016. Arch Dis Child 103:A22
34. Tomasz A (1997) Antibiotic resistance in Streptococcus pneumoniae. Clin Infect Dis 24 (Supplement_1):S85–S88
35. Oligbu G, Collins S, Sheppard CL, Fry NK, Slack M, Borrow R et al (2017) Childhood deaths attributable to invasive pneumococcal disease in England and Wales, 2006–2014. Clin Infect Dis 65(2):308–314
36. Ladhani SN, Slack MP, Andrews NJ, Waight PA, Borrow R, Miller E (2013) Invasive pneumococcal disease after routine pneumococcal conjugate vaccination in children England and Wales. Emerg Infect Dis 19(1):61
37. Singleton RJ, Hennessy TW, Bulkow LR, Hammitt LL, Zulz T, Hurlburt DA et al (2007) Invasive pneumococcal disease caused by nonvaccine serotypes among Alaska native children with high levels of 7-valent pneumococcal conjugate vaccine coverage. JAMA 297 (16):1784–1792
38. Centers for Disease Control and Prevention (2013) Active bacterial core surveillance report, emerging infections program network, streptococcus pneumoniae, 2011. Accessed 12 May 2018
39. Nuorti JP, Whitney CG (2010) Prevention of pneumococcal disease among infants and children: use of 13-valent pneumococcal conjugate vaccine and 23-valent pneumococcal polysaccharide vaccine: recommendations of the advisory committee on immunization practices (ACIP). Department of Health and Human Services, Centers for Disease Control and Prevention. MMWR Recomm Rep 59 (RR-11):1–18
40. Van Hoek AJ, Andrews N, Waight PA, Stowe J, Gates P, George R et al (2012) The effect of underlying clinical conditions on the risk of developing invasive pneumococcal disease in England. J Infect 65(1):17–24

41. Bliss SJ, O'Brien KL, Janoff EN, Cotton MF, Musoke P, Coovadia H et al (2008) The evidence for using conjugate vaccines to protect HIV-infected children against pneumococcal disease. Lancet Infect Dis 8:67–80
42. Nunes MC, Von Gottberg A, de Gouveia L et al (2011) The impact of antiretroviral treatment on the burden of invasive pneumococcal disease in South African children: a time series analysis. AIDS 25(4):453–462
43. Oligbu G, Collins S, Sheppard C, Fry N, Dick M, Streetly A, Ladhani S. (2018). Risk of Invasive Pneumococcal Disease in Children with Sickle Cell Disease in England: A National Observational Cohort Study, 2010–2015. *Archives of disease in childhood*, 103(7): 643–647

Chapter 18

The Epidemiology and Biostatistics of Pneumococcus

Godwin Oligbu, Norman K. Fry, and Shamez N. Ladhani

Abstract

Invasive infections caused by *Streptococcus pneumoniae*, such as pneumonia, meningitis, and bacteremia, are a major cause of morbidity and mortality in young children and older adults worldwide. The introduction of pneumococcal conjugate vaccines into national childhood immunization programs has led to large and sustained reductions in the incidence of invasive pneumococcal disease across all age groups. Here we describe the epidemiology and biostatistics of pneumococcal disease as well as the impact of vaccination on the burden of pneumococcal disease globally.

Key words *Streptococcus pneumoniae*, Invasive pneumococcal disease, Pneumococcal conjugate vaccine, Public health, Surveillance

1 Introduction

Diseases caused by the pneumococcus are a major public health problem, both in terms of the large burden of non-invasive diseases such as otitis media, sinusitis and non-bacteremic pneumonia, as well as the poor outcomes associated with more severe invasive infections including meningitis and septicemia [1–4]. Polysaccharide vaccines against the pneumococcus have been available for several decades, but it was the licensure of the pneumococcal conjugate vaccine (PCV) for infants and young children in 2000 that led to rapid and sustained declines in invasive pneumococcal disease (IPD) in countries with established national immunization programs and high vaccine uptake. Here we describe the epidemiology and biostatistics of the pneumococcus as well as the impact of vaccination on the burden of pneumococcal disease globally.

2 Material and Methods

2.1 Search Strategy

A search strategy was undertaken to define the burden of invasive pneumococcal disease and the impact of vaccination in countries

Federico Iovino (ed.), *Streptococcus pneumoniae: Methods and Protocols*, Methods in Molecular Biology, vol. 1968, https://doi.org/10.1007/978-1-4939-9199-0_18,

with established PCV immunization programs. We searched MEDLINE, EMBASE, and the Cochrane library from first January 2000 to 30th April 2016, as well as the ISI web of knowledge, to identify relevant articles and conference proceedings. The medical subject headings (MeSH) terms used included "invasive pneumococcal disease," "pneumococcal polysaccharide vaccine," "pneumococcal conjugate vaccines," "Streptococcus pneumoniae," "pneumococcus," "PCV7," "PCV10," and "PCV13." We included studies published in English language. In addition, we screened reference lists of selected papers to retrieve relevant studies.

Studies were eligible for inclusion if they reported vaccine impact and effectiveness from observational studies, case–control studies and surveillance databases. The title and abstract of all identified publications were screened, and full articles of included publications were retrieved and reviewed for eligibility. Eligible studies were then assessed according to the Reporting Items for Systematic Reviews and Meta-analyses (PRISMA) statement for the conduct and reporting of systematic reviews.

3 Findings

3.1 The Burden of Pneumococcal Disease

Pneumococcal disease remains a leading cause of vaccine-preventable child illness and death despite continuing reductions in both overall childhood mortality and pneumonia deaths. Unlike invasive pneumococcal disease (IPD) where there are established surveillance systems, the overall burden of non-invasive pneumococcal disease has been difficult to measure, especially the attribution of the pneumococcus to community-acquired bacterial pneumonia (CAP) where the pathogen responsible is rarely identified. It is estimated globally that there were 120 million episodes of non-bacteremic pneumonia in 2010 in developing countries, resulting in 1.3 million deaths in children younger than 5 years [5]. Before the introduction of pneumococcal conjugate vaccines (PCVs) in low income countries, of the estimated 8.8 million global annual deaths amongst children <5 years of age in 2008, nearly half a million deaths were caused by pneumococcal infections in HIV-negative children [6]. Children and adults with underlying comorbidities have a much higher risk of serious pneumococcal disease and death [7]. The highest burden of pneumonia deaths is in Africa and Southeast Asia, which together account for almost 1 million of the estimated 1.3 million pneumonia deaths worldwide in children under 5 years of age [5], and a significant proportion of those deaths could arguably have been prevented through vaccination.

The incidence of IPD in children aged <5 years is also much higher in developing countries than industrialized countries for a number of reasons, including malnutrition, poverty, and overcrowding. Disease incidence in developing countries is generally underestimated due to inadequate facility to establish diagnosis, self-medication, and poor surveillance systems. For example, in South Africa, prior to PCV introduction, the incidence of IPD in <2 years among HIV uninfected children was 28.6/100,000, while in Gambia the incidence was estimated to be 253/100,000 in a similar age-group [8]. In developed countries, too, the reported incidence in children <5 years old in the pre-PCV era has been variable, ranging from 17.1 to 94.7 cases/100,000 child-years, with the highest incidence in North-America and lowest in European countries [9].

In adults, the annual incidence of IPD ranges from 15 to 49 per 100,000 in North America, whereas in Europe, during the same period, the rates ranged from 11 to 27 per 100,000 [10–12]. *S. pneumoniae* is the most common cause of CAP in adults. The overall incidence of CAP rises rapidly with increasing age, with estimated rates ranging from 18.2 per 1000 person-years in people aged 65–69 years, to 52.3 per 1000 person-years in those aged over 85 years [13]. Case fatality from CAP also increases with age, being 2.2% vs. 10.3% in these two age-groups respectively, in a large Spanish cohort [14]. Amongst those with underlying co-morbidity, those with predisposing factors for IPD and elderly patients with severe CAP requiring mechanical ventilation had case fatality rates of more than 50% [15]. Robust data on the burden of pneumococcal disease in adults and elderly people in developing countries, especially relating to pneumonia, are lacking [16]. Generally, adults with underlying comorbidities and older adults are more vulnerable to serious bacterial infection and are also less likely to develop robust immune responses to vaccination [17]. The ageing human population, especially in developed countries, poses a major challenge and will lead to a rise in the healthcare and economic burden for pneumococcal diseases worldwide. In the USA, in 2004, it was estimated that the direct healthcare costs of pneumococcal disease totaled $3.5 billion [18]. A similar study in Europe estimated that the total healthcare costs for CAP could be as high as $11.7 billion annually, with one-third related to indirect costs, such as loss of working days [19]. It was, therefore, clear that a long-lasting solution was needed to curb the burden of pneumococcal disease in developing and industrialized countries. In 2000, PCV7 was introduced in the USA and later adopted in the national immunization program of many other countries.

3.2 PCVs' Impact on Invasive Pneumococcal Disease

The introduction of PCV7 into national childhood immunization programs led to a significant and sustained decline in IPD caused by PCV7 serotypes in countries with high childhood vaccine uptake, not only in the vaccinated cohorts but also in older unvaccinated cohorts because of indirect (herd) protection [20].

Unlike the polysaccharide vaccines, PCV are highly immunogenic across all age groups including young infants; they induce a T-cell-mediated immune response which leads to an IgG-mediated antibody response and longer-lasting immune response, induction of immune memory and boosting with subsequent vaccine doses, and prevention of carriage in the nasopharynx of immunized individuals. Nasopharyngeal carriage among infants and toddlers is an important driver of pneumococcal transmission in the household and the wider community [21]. PCV impact on carriage reduction was recently summarized in a systematic review [22]. However, overall carriage rate in children have remained unchanged because PCV7 serotypes were replaced with non-PCV7 serotypes in carriage and, consequently, in disease [23]. Despite a small increase in serotype replacement disease due to non-PCV7 serotypes, overall IPD rates, especially in developed countries with high vaccine uptake, have declined significantly across all age groups and especially in the vaccinated cohort [24]. In the UK, for example, an overall reduction of 37% compared to the pre-PCV7 period was observed across all age-groups through a combination of direct and indirect (herd) protection [25].

Other countries that introduced PCV7 also observed similar rapid reductions in overall and PCV7-serotype IPD, with variable extent of replacement disease [26–29]. In the review published by Myint et al (2013) on the impact of PCV7 on IPD in Europe, vaccine-type IPD reduction ranged from 39.9% in Spain to 99.1% in the USA with a median rate reduction of 90.1% [30]. These countries also observed replacement with non-vaccine serotypes, in both carriage and disease, following the successful implementation of PCV7 [31–34]. The impact of PCVs on pneumococcal meningitis in countries with established pneumococcal immunization programs has been variable, with some countries reporting significant reductions after PCV7 introduction and others reporting no change, or a decline only after PCV13 introduction [35–40].

The main replacing serotypes varied in different countries but some of the emerging serotypes were consistently common, including serotypes 6C, 19A, 22F, 15, and 33 [41–43]. Replacement disease with serotype 19A was a particular problem in many parts of the world, but especially in the USA, because this serotype was associated with resistance to multiple antibiotics [44, 45]. Since PCV7 licensure, two higher valent vaccines (PCV10 and PCV13) were licensed after they were shown to elicit an adequate immune response against all the vaccine serotypes with demonstrated non-inferiority against the serotypes they have in common with PCV7 [46].

Globally, the introduction of higher-valent PCVs, including those countries with established PCV7 programs, has led to additional reductions in overall IPD rates, albeit with serotype replacement due to new emerging serotypes in carriage and disease. Currently, the 10 most common serotypes causing IPD in Europe include (in order of frequency) 8, 3, 22F, 12F, 19A, 9N, 7F, 15A, 33F, and 10A, accounting for 62% of serotyped isolates. Of the cases in children under 5 years of age, 72% were caused by a serotype not included in any PCV. Among cases aged 65 years and over, 71% were caused by a PPV23 serotype, and 32% were caused by a PCV13 serotype [47]. As expected, the overall decrease in IPD incidence has been eroded in part by the increasing incidence of replacement IPD due to non-vaccine serotypes, especially in the elderly.

3.3 PCVs' Impact on Pneumonia and Death

Prior to PCV introduction, a randomised controlled trial (RCT) conducted in the Gambia using a 9-valent PCV (PCV9) in the early 2000s found that the vaccine reduced all-cause mortality by 16% (3–28%) [31]. Following this trial, the WHO estimated that global use of PCVs would reduce mortality due to pneumonia in children by 25–30% [48]. Subsequently, a recent global burden assessment found that about half of all fatal lower respiratory tract infections (LRTIs) are caused by pneumococcus and the majority of cases are, thus, potentially vaccine-preventable [49]. However, a systematic review and meta-analysis of randomized controlled studies did not find PCVs to have a statistically significant effect on death due to pneumonia [50, 51]. The magnitude of serotype replacement in pneumococcal pneumonia is not known and will be difficult to measure because of diagnostic, methodological, and surveillance challenges. In particular, it is difficult to disentangle contribution of vaccine-related changes to natural fluctuations in serotype dynamics in different populations.

3.4 PCVs' Impact on Antibiotic Resistance

The impact of PCVs on antibiotic resistance among pneumococcal strains causing IPD has varied in different part of the world. In 1998, prior to PCV use, the Centre for Disease Control and Prevention reported that 24% of strains associated with IPD were nonsusceptible to penicillin and that serotypes 6B, 9V, 14, 19F, and 23F accounted for 78% of penicillin nonsusceptible strains [52]. During the PCV7 era, serotypes 7F and 19A, among others, emerged mainly through clonal expansion as the most common replacing serotypes causing meningitis in Europe and the USA [25, 53, 54]. Unlike the UK, however, the emerging serotype 19A strains in several countries, including France and the USA, exhibited high rates of resistance to multiple antibiotics [55, 56]. In South Africa, two years after PCV7 introduction, vaccine effectiveness against all-serotype multidrug-resistant IPD was 96% (95% CI, 62%, 100%) among HIV-uninfected children [57]. Following three years of PCV use, penicillin nonsusceptible IPD rates declined by 47% (95% CI: 38%, 55%) in South African children <2 years; this was predominately due to a decline in the proportion of penicillin nonsusceptible PCV7 serotypes from 70% of isolates in 2009 to 47% of isolates in 2012 [58].

Following the introduction of PCV13, many countries have demonstrated significant large reductions in IPD caused by the additional PCV13 serotypes, including serotype 19A and the antimicrobial resistant clones [59–61]. However, this serotype continues to circulate and cause invasive disease despite widespread use of PCV13 in industrialized countries with established immunization programs [62].

3.5 Pneumococcal Polysaccharide Vaccines

PPV23 immunization offers protection against 11 additional pneumococcal serotypes compared to PCV13. Many countries continue to recommend PPV23 for high-risk individuals and older adults from 65 years of age [63, 64]. However, there is controversy regarding PPV23 effectiveness and duration of protection, especially against non-invasive pneumococcal disease [65], and a hypothetical risk of PPV23-induced immunological hyporesponsiveness [66]. Because of the changing epidemiology of IPD, especially serotype replacement disease following the successful implementation of PCVs into national immunization programs [54], offering PPV23 to high-risk individuals is likely to become more important in the coming years. The UK and other countries have reported large increase in IPD due to serotypes that are included in PPV23 and not in PCV13 since PCV13 replaced PCV7 in the national immunization programme [25]. A pneumococcal conjugate vaccine covering the additional serotypes that are only included in PPV23 would be very welcome.

4 Conclusions

S. pneumoniae is a major public health problem with significant burden to global health. In light of the efforts to reduce the burden of IPD worldwide, routine immunization with pneumococcal conjugate vaccines was introduced at different times in different countries. To date, 139 countries have introduced a PCV in their infant immunization programme [67]. Widespread availability of PCVs has reduced the burden of IPD substantially in children under 5 years of age, from over 800,000 annual deaths before PCV introduction to 541,000 deaths in 2008 [6, 7]. Additional impact has been observed in adult because of herd effects but to a variable extent. The benefits of the current PCVs is likely to decline in the developed countries because of serotype replacement disease, but will continue to have a major impact in developing countries where most pneumococcal deaths still occur. With variable increases in replacement disease due to different serotypes, increased collaboration between countries and a more global surveillance are essential. Meanwhile, alternative strategies such as protein-based serotype-independent will be needed to curb the problem of serotype replacement disease.

References

1. Russel F, Sanderson C, Temple B, Mulholand K (2011) Global review of the distribution of pneumococcal disease by age and region. World Health Organization, Geneva, Switzerland. http://www.who.int/immunization/sage/6_Russel_review_age_specific_epidemiology_PCV_schedules_session_novl 1.pdf. 2011.Nov
2. Drijkoningen JJ, Rhode GG (2014) Pneumococcal infection in adults: burden of disease. Clin Microbiol Infect 20:45–51
3. Advisory Committee on Immunization Practices (2000) Preventing pneumococcal disease among infants and young children. Recommendations of the Advisory Committee on Immunization Practices (ACIP). MMWR Recomm Rep 49(RR-9):1–35
4. Butler JC, Schuchat A (1999) Epidemiology of pneumococcal infections in the elderly. Drugs Aging 15(Suppl 1):11–19
5. Walker CL, Rudan I, Liu L, Nair H, Theodoratou E, Bhutta ZA et al (2013) Global burden of childhood pneumonia and diarrhoea. Lancet 381(9875):1405–1416
6. World Health Organization (2008) Estimated Hib and pneumococcal deaths for children under 5 years of age. http://www.who.int/immunization/monitoring_surveillance/burden/estimates/Pneumo_hib/en/. Accessed 12 May
7. O'Brien KL, Wolfson LJ, Watt JP, Henkle E, Deloria-Knoll M, McCall N et al (2009) Burden of disease caused by Streptococcus pneumoniae in children younger than 5 years: global estimates. Lancet 374(9693):893–902
8. Mackenzie GA, Hill PC, Jeffries DJ, Hossain I, Uchendu U, Ameh D et al (2016) Effect of the introduction of pneumococcal conjugate vaccination on invasive pneumococcal disease in The Gambia: a population-based surveillance study. Lancet Infect Dis 16(6):703–711
9. Izurieta P, Bahety P, Adegbola R, Clarke C, Hoet B (2018) Public health impact of pneumococcal conjugate vaccine infant immunization programs: assessment of invasive pneumococcal disease burden and serotype distribution. Expert Rev Vaccines 17(6):479–493
10. Kyaw MH, Christie P, Clarke SC, Mooney JD, Ahmed S, Jones IG et al (2003) Invasive pneumococcal disease in Scotland, 1999–2001: use of record linkage to explore associations between patients and disease in relation to future vaccination policy. Clin Infect Dis 37:1283–1291
11. Reinert RR, Haupts S, van der LM HC, Cil MY, Al-Lahham A et al (2005) Invasive pneumococcal disease in adults in North-Rhine Westphalia, Germany, 2001–2003. Clin Microbiol Infect 11:985–991
12. Lynch JP, Zhanel GG (2009) Streptococcus pneumoniae: epidemiology, risk factors, and strategies for prevention. Semin Respir Crit Care Med 30:189–209
13. Jackson ML, Neuzil KM, Thomson WW et al (2004) The burden of community-acquired pneumonia in seniors: results of a population-based study. Clin Infect Dis 39:1642–1650
14. Vila-Corcoles A, Ochoa-Gondar O, Llor C, Rodríguez T, Gómez A (2005) Protective effect of pneumococcal vaccine against death by pneumonia in elderly subjects. Eur Respir J 26(6):1086–1091
15. El-Solh AA, Sikka P, Ramadan F, Davies J (2001) Etiology of severe pneumonia in the very elderly. Am J Respir Crit Care Med 163 (3 Pt 1):645–651
16. Maimaiti N, Ahmed Z, Isa ZM, Ghazi HF, Aljunid S (2013) Clinical burden of invasive pneumococcal disease in selected developing countries. Value Health Reg Issues 2 (2):259–263
17. Weycker D, Strutton D, Edelsberg J, Sato R, Jackson LA (2010) Clinical and economic burden of pneumococcal disease in older US adults. Vaccine 28:4955–4960
18. Huang SS, Johnson KM, Ray GT et al (2011) Healthcare utilization and cost of pneumococcal disease in the United States. Vaccine 29:3398–3412
19. Gibson GJ, Loddenkemper R, Sibille Y, European Respiratory Society/European Lung Foundation (2003) Lung Health in Europe Facts and Figures. ERSJ, Sheffield
20. Davis SM, Deloria-Knoll M, Kassa HT, O'Brien KL (2013) Impact of pneumococcal conjugate vaccines on nasopharyngeal carriage and invasive disease among unvaccinated people: review of evidence on indirect effects. Vaccine 32:133–145
21. Hennessy TW, Singleton RJ, Bulkow LR et al (2005) Impact of heptavalent pneumococcal conjugate vaccine on invasive disease,

antimicrobial resistance and colonization in Alaska Natives: progress towards elimination of a health disparity. Vaccine 23:5464–5473

22. Cohen R, Levy C, Bingen E, Bonnet E, Koskas M, Attal S, et al (2011) Impact of 13-valent pneumococcal conjugate vaccine (PCV13) on nasopharyngeal (NP) flora in children with acute otitis media (AOM). In: Presented at the 51st ICAAC, September 17–20, 2011, Chicago, USA
23. Conklin L, Loo JD, Kirk J, Fleming-Dutra KE, Deloria Knoll M, Park DE et al (2014) Systematic review of the effect of pneumococcal conjugate vaccine dosing schedules on vaccine-type invasive pneumococcal disease among young children. Pediatr Infect Dis J 33(Suppl 2 Optimum Dosing of Pneumococcal Conjugate Vaccine For Infants 0 A Landscape Analysis of Evidence Supporting Different Schedules):S109–S118
24. Kaplan SL, Barson WJ, Lin PL, Romero JR, Bradley JS, Tan TQ et al (2013) Early trends for invasive pneumococcal infections in children after the introduction of the 13-valent pneumococcal conjugate vaccine. Pediatr Infect Dis J 32:203–207
25. Waight PA, Andrews NJ, Ladhani SN, Sheppard CL, Slack MPE, Miller E (2015) Effect of the 13-valent pneumococcal conjugate vaccine on invasive pneumococcal disease in England and Wales 4 years after its introduction: an observational cohort study. Lancet Infect Dis 15(5):535–543
26. Gilmour R, Holland R, Kampen R, Brown M, Gilbert L, Hogg G et al (2008) Invasive pneumococcal disease in Australia, 2006. Commun Dis Intell 32(1):18–30
27. Kellner JD, Church DL, MacDonald J, Tyrrell GJ, Scheifele D (2005) Progress in the prevention of pneumococcal infection. Can Med Assoc J 173(10):1149–1151
28. Zangeneh TT, Baracco G, Al-Tawfiq JA (2011) Impact of conjugate pneumococcal vaccines on the changing epidemiology of pneumococcal infections. Expert Rev Vaccines 10 (3):345–353
29. World Health Organization position paper - Pneumococcal conjugate vaccine for childhood immunization (2007) WHO position paper. Wkly Epidemiol Rec 82(12):93–104
30. Myint TT, Madhava H, Balmer P, Christopoulou D, Attal S, Menegas D et al (2013) The impact of 7-valent pneumococcal conjugate vaccine on invasive pneumococcal disease: a literature review. Adv Ther 30 (2):127–151
31. Miller E, Andrews NJ, Waight PA, Slack MPE, George RC (2011) Herd immunity and serotype replacement 4 years after seven-valent pneumococcal conjugate vaccination in England and Wales: an observational cohort study. Lancet Infect Dis 11(10):760–768
32. Weinberger DM, Malley RLM (2011) Serotype replacement in disease after pneumococcal vaccination. Lancet 378(9807):1962–1973
33. Singleton RJ, Hennessy TW, Bulkow LR, Hammitt LL, Zulz T, Hurlburt DA et al (2007) Invasive pneumococcal disease caused by nonvaccine serotypes among Alaska native children with high levels of 7-valent pneumococcal conjugate vaccine coverage. JAMA 297 (16):1784–1792
34. Park SY, Van Beneden CA, Pilishvili T, Martin M, Facklam RR, Whitney CG (2010) Invasive pneumococcal infections among vaccinated children in the United States active bacterial core surveillance team. J Pediatr 158 (3):478–483.e2
35. Ben-Shimol S, Givon-Lavi N, Grisaru-Soen G, Megged O, Greenberg D, Dagan R (2017) Comparative incidence dynamics and serotypes of meningitis, bacteremic pneumonia and other-IPD in young children in the PCV era: Insights from Israeli surveillance studies. Vaccine 36(36):5477–5484
36. Alari A, Chaussade H, Domenech De Cellès M, Le Fouler L, Varon E, Opatowski L et al (2016) Impact of pneumococcal conjugate vaccines on pneumococcal meningitis cases in France between 2001 and 2014: a time series analysis. BMC Med 14(1):211
37. Hsu HE, Shutt KA, Moore MR, Beall BW, Bennett NM, Craig AS et al (2009) Effect of pneumococcal conjugate vaccine on pneumococcal meningitis. N Engl J Med 360 (3):244–256
38. Ruiz-Contreras J, Picazo J, Casado-Flores J, Baquero-Artigao F, Hernández-Sampelayo T, HERACLES STUDY GROUP et al (2017) Impact of 13-valent pneumococcal conjugate vaccine on pneumococcal meningitis in children. Vaccine 35(35 Pt B):4646–4651
39. Tsai CJ, Griffin MR, Nuorti JP, Grijalva GC (2008) Changing epidemiology of pneumococcal meningitis after introduction of pneumococcal conjugate vaccine in the United States. Clin Infect Dis 46(11):1664–1672
40. Olarte L, Barson WJ, Barson RM, Lin PL, Romero JR, Tan TQ et al (2015) Impact of the 13-valent pneumococcal conjugate vaccine on pneumococcal meningitis in US children. Clin Infect Dis 61(5):767–775

41. Jacobs M (2008) Antimicrobial-resistant streptococcus pneumoniae: trends and management. Expert Rev Anti-Infect Ther 6 (5):619–635
42. Park IH, Moore MR, Treanor JJ, Pelton SI, Pilishvili T, Beall B et al (2008) Active bacteria core surveillance team. Differential effects of pneumococcal vaccines against serotypes 6A and 6C. J Infect Dis 198(12):1818–1822
43. Pelton SI, Huot H, Finkelstein JA, Bishop CJ, Hsu KK, Kellenberg J et al (2007) Emergence of 19A as virulent and multidrug resistant Pneumococcus in Massachusetts following universal immunization of infants with pneumococcal conjugate vaccine. Pediatr Infect Dis J 26(6):468–472
44. Pai R, Moore MR, Pilishvili T, Gertz RE, Whitney CG, Beall B (2005) Postvaccine genetic structure of Streptococcus pneumoniae serotype 19A from children in the United States. J Infect Dis 192(11):1988–1995
45. Yildirim I, Stevenson A, Hsu KK, Pelton SI (2012) Evolving picture of invasive pneumococcal disease in Massachusetts children: a comparison of disease in 2007–2009 with earlier periods. Pediatr Infect Dis J 31 (10):1016–1021
46. Vanderkooi OG, Scheifele DW, Girgenti D, Halperin SA, Patterson SD, Gruber WC et al (2012) Safety and immunogenicity of a 13-valent pneumococcal conjugate vaccine in healthy infants and toddlers given with routine pediatric vaccinations in Canada. Pediatr Infect Dis J 31(1):72–77
47. European Centre for Disease Prevention and Control (2017) Invasive pneumococcal disease. Stockholm. https://ecdc.europa.eu/en/publications-data/invasive-pneumococcal-disease-annual-epidemiological-report-2017. Accessed 12 May 2018
48. World Health Organization, UNICEF (2013) Ending preventable child deaths from pneumonia and diarrhoea by 2025: The integrated Global Action Plan for Pneumonia and Diarrhoea (GAPPD)
49. Troeger C, Forouzanfar M, Rao PC, Khalil I, Brown A, Reiner RC Jr et al (2017) Estimates of global, regional, and national morbidity, mortality, and aetiologies of diarrhoeal diseases: a systematic analysis for the Global Burden of Disease Study 2015. Lancet Infect Dis 3099(17):1–40
50. Lucero M, Dulalia V, Nillos L, Williams G, Parreño R, Nohynek H et al (2009) Pneumococcal conjugate vaccines for preventing vaccine-type invasive pneumococcal disease and X-ray defined pneumonia in children less than two years of age. Cochrane Database Syst Rev 4:CD004977
51. Ewald H, Briel M, Vuichard D, Kreutle V, Zhydkov A, Gloy V (2016) The clinical effectiveness of pneumococcal conjugate vaccines: a systematic review and metaanalysis of randomized controlled trials. Dtsch Arztebl Int 113 (9):139–146
52. Whitney CG, Farley MM, Hadler J, Harrison LH, Lexau C, Reingold A et al (2000) Active bacterial core surveillance program of the emerging infections program network. Increasing prevalence of multidrug-resistant streptococcus pneumoniae in the United States. N Engl J Med 343(26):1917–1924
53. Richter SS, Heilmann KP, Dohrn CL, Riahi F, Diekema DJ, Doern GV (2013) Pneumococcal serotypes before and after introduction of conjugate vaccines, United States, 1999–2011. Emerg Infect Dis 19(7):1074–1083
54. Hanquet G, Kissling E, Fenoll A, George R, Lepoutre A, Lernout T et al (2010) Pneumococcal serotypes in children in 4 European countries. Emerg Infect Dis 16(9):1428–1439
55. Janoir C, Lepoutre A, Gutmann L, Varon E (2016) Insight into resistance phenotypes of emergent non 13-valent pneumococcal conjugate vaccine type pneumococci isolated from invasive disease after 13-valent Pneumococcal conjugate vaccine implementation in France. Open Forum Infect Dis 3(1):ofw020
56. Mahjoub-Messai F, Doit C, Koeck JL, Billard T, Evrard B, Bidet P et al (2009) Population snapshot of Streptococcus pneumoniae serotype 19A isolates before and after introduction of seven-valent pneumococcal vaccination for French children. J Clin Microbiol 47 (3):837–840
57. Cohen C, von Mollendorf C, de Gouveia L, Naidoo N, Meiring S, Quan V et al (2014) Effectiveness of 7-valent pneumococcal conjugate vaccine against invasive pneumococcal disease in HIV-infected and -uninfected children in South Africa: a matched case-control study. Clin Infect Dis 59:808–818
58. Von Gottberg A, de Gouveia L, Tempia S, Quan V, Meiring S, Von Mollendorf C et al (2014) Effects of vaccination on invasive pneumococcal disease in South Africa. N Engl J Med 371(20):1889–1899
59. Moore MR, Link-Gelles R, Schaffner W et al (2016) Effectiveness of 13- valent pneumococcal conjugate vaccine for prevention of invasive pneumococcal disease in children in the USA: a matched case- control study. Lancet Respir Med 4:399–406

60. Isturiz R, Sings HL, Hilton B, Arguedas A, Reinert RR, Jodar L (2017) Streptococcus pneumoniae serotype 19A: worldwide epidemiology. Expert Rev Vaccines 16 (10):1007–1027
61. Gaviria-Agudelo CL, Jordan-Villegas A, Garcia C, McCracken GH Jr (2017) The effect of 13-valent pneumococcal conjugate vaccine on the serotype distribution and antibiotic resistance profiles in children with invasive pneumococcal disease. J Pediatr Infect Dis Soc 6(3):253–259
62. Balsells E, Guillot L, Nair H, Kyaw MH (2017) Serotype distribution of Streptococcus pneumoniae causing invasive disease in children in the post-PCV era: A systematic review and meta-analysis. PLoS One 12(5):e0177113
63. Tomczyk S, Bennett NM, Stoecker C, Gierke R, Moore MR, Whitney CG, Centre for Disease Control and Prevention (CDC) et al (2014) Use of 13-valent pneumococcal conjugate vaccine and 23-valent pneumococcal polysaccharide vaccine among adults aged ≥65 years: recommendations of the Advisory Committee on Immunization Practices (ACIP). Morb Mortal Wkly Rep 63:822–825
64. Persons I (2013) Use of 13-valent pneumococcal conjugate vaccine and 23-valent pneumococcal polysaccharide vaccine among children aged 6–18 years with immunocompromising conditions: recommendations of the Advisory Committee on Immunization Practices (ACIP). Morb Mortal Wkly Rep 62(25):521
65. Huss A, Scott P, Stuck AE, Trotter C, Egger M (2009) Efficacy of pneumococcal vaccination in adults: a meta-analysis. Can Med Assoc J 180:48–58
66. Poolman J, Borrow R (2011) Hyporesponsiveness and its clinical implications after vaccination with polysaccharide or glycoconjugate vaccines. Expert Rev Vaccines 10:307–322
67. VIEW-hub [Internet]. PCV: Current vaccine intro status. [Cited 2018 May12]. http://view-hub.org/viz/

INDEX

Federico Iovino (ed.), *Streptococcus pneumoniae: Methods and Protocols*, Methods in Molecular Biology, vol. 1968,
https://doi.org/10.1007/978-1-4939-9199-0,

H

I

L

M

N

P

R

S

T

U

W

Z

MIX
Papier aus verantwortungsvollen Quellen
Paper from responsible sources
FSC® C105338

If you have any concerns about our products,
you can contact us on
ProductSafety@springernature.com

In case Publisher is established outside the EU,
the EU authorized representative is:
Springer Nature Customer Service Center GmbH
Europaplatz 3, 69115 Heidelberg, Germany

Printed by Libri Plureos GmbH
in Hamburg, Germany